Gastric Band and
BEYOND

Maximise your weight loss

Mrs Sharon E. Bates;
Dr Simon J.W. Monkhouse

authorHOUSE®

AuthorHouse™ UK Ltd.
500 Avebury Boulevard
Central Milton Keynes, MK9 2BE
www.authorhouse.co.uk
Phone: 08001974150

First published by AuthorHouse 12/27/2010

ISBN: 978-1-4567-7174-4 (sc)

CONTENTS

Chapter 1

MY STORY...

I consider myself fortunate to work with a wonderfully complex and amazing population of bariatric patients.

Difficulties, complaints, personal processes are all part of life. To bear witness to an adult's personal change journey of weight loss is, to me, such a privilege. I was a midwife for many years and this weight loss journey can be as amazing to witness as being present at a birth.

Weight loss surgery

I wonder why many feel that having surgery to aid weight loss is the 'easy way out'. In reality it is far from easy and most certainly not, 'the easy way out'.

The journey of weight loss, weight loss surgery and personal change and growth for me is one that never ceases to amaze me and this book, I hope, will explore some of the issues that are less recognised.

In 2000, weight loss surgery was far from well known or commercially 'sexy'. A few surgeons in the UK had a growing private practice and even fewer were able to offer gastric banding or bypass within the NHS.

My battle began from the inception of the idea of having 'a band'. The hurdles of judgement, ignorance, admonishment and mocking disbelief were there from the seed of desire to have something to help me escape from my own adipose. I sought help and advice. Sadly, I received professional disparaging disapproval as I wanted to walk on unknown ground.

I was desperate and death was a far more appealing option than getting fatter and fatter and, even fatter.

The physical metamorphosis over the years following gastric banding has been exciting, incredible and also unbelievable to me. Emotionally and physically the journey, as with us all, continues.

I honestly believed at the time that it was simply 'a band' put around the top part of my stomach. I thought it would work and I thought once I had lost my weight everything would be easy. I would be 'cured' once and for all of my life-long, all consuming battle with being too fat.

I had very skewed understanding of food and eating.

Food was something I feared as it equated to weight gain. Eating was something I enjoyed. I had a buzz and sense of contentment. I longed for the temporary effect and yet loathed what I saw to be the inevitable permanent impact. Yet food was a consistent factor in my life and a very good friend.

When I had lost size, I gradually lost the sense of needing to judge myself by my size. Who I am is no longer closely associated to my size.

Admittedly, at times I was (and am still) angry that I simply couldn't eat what I wanted to, either in quantity or in junk like quality.

I honestly believed that once I'd got 'there' – to Shangri-La – I wouldn't have to think about losing weight. When I was moaning that I couldn't eat anything and not gain weight my 'size 10' daughters said to me …. "but Mummy it is hard work to stay slim."

Then it 'clicked'. I realised after four years as a 'banded person' … the journey never ends and now, even more years forward I say … the journey never ends. The banding journey is simply that, a journey, not a destination.

From approximately 2006, weight loss surgery in the UK became a 'sexy subject'. Magazines, TV presenter stories and radio programmes have been singing the praises of the 'magic wand' surgery to attain 'slimness'. Slimness itself being what for some equates to acceptance by self and others in today's society.

This book is hopefully a brief explanation of what the surgery entails but also an exploration of the other issues around weight loss. I want to touch areas that so many have tried to express in a consultation setting and feeling they are the only ones…but …they're not.

Me, myself, my shape and size …

I was born in the mid 1950's. This meant that my generation was generally free from wartime rationing. I guess we are probably the first generation to experience food as readily available and somewhat unlimited in supply.

I remember the first birthday party where we had 'ice cream' with our jelly, the excitement of having a 'freezer' at home and the resulting foods that were marketed to fill it. Swiftly came more and more 'fast foods', 'junk foods', 'ready-made meals in a pack' and marketing strategies that resulted in me choosing to buy and eat more.

Food was, and still is, a wonderful commodity to me.

As a child I would explore our garden, pull radishes from the ground, wipe them on my thick grey gym knickers then eat them. I would dig potatoes with a friend, build a small bonfire and bake them 'secretly' in the garden. I would eat my Easter eggs in one day; my brother would store his for months. I guess he must have known I stole from his secret tin though ....

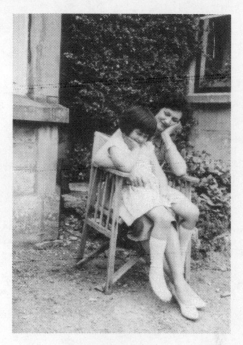

Me aged about 6

As many parents in the 1960's my mother made most of my clothes. I was a 'problem'. 'Chubby patterns' were the only dress patterns that she could use that would fit. It meant more fabric and more fabric was expensive. My friends could wear jeans but they simply didn't make jeans in my size. So, I felt left out running in the fields in a skirt or home made shorts. Even school uniform was too small and had to be specially ordered.

I wonder, how many of us in that generation were pulled

from a class to 'be weighed' by the school nurse? How many of us had 'special meals' at school? How many of us felt embarrassed by – 'segregation of the size' in gym, Rounders, netball but thankfully not hockey. Although my brother would say they only selected me to block the goal rather than because I was a goal keeper.

At about 10 yrs old, I was taken to the Bristol Children's Hospital. Everyone was concerned that I was 'so fat'. The diagnosis and treatment was that it was 'puppy fat', I was 'pre-pubescent' and to stick to a diet of 1,000 calories a day.

By the age of 12 years, I was an expert on counting calories, food deprivation and judging my self-worth against how 'good' or how 'bad' I had been on a diet.

You must have been enormous, I hear some say.

11 stone at aged 11years, 5 foot 4 inches - a Body Mass Index (BMI) of 26.4

This BMI is today deemed as 'overweight'. Not obese and not morbidly obese. However, in comparison with the then 'norm' I was very fat. I felt elephantine and had been placed in a position of 'fatness'. It was later to become a self fulfilling prophecy.

Late in 1970s came John Denver, Fondue parties, chilli-con-carne, cheesecake and growing numbers of supermarkets.

Chocolate bars and bags of crisps had overnight 'growth spurts' on the shelves and big portions became an endorsement of excellence. Small became regular, regular became large, large became super large.

I reflected the trend and increased in size. However, I did not come with the endorsement of excellence.

At size 16/18 I was not the average size for a British female.

In 1979 I was to go with a group of friends to the USA. I was challenged by my family – I was too fat to travel. Would I fit into the seat? How can I possibly go looking like 'this' ~ 'this' meant 'fat'.

Of course, when I got to the USA, my then size 16/18 was slim in comparison with the population, my size 10/12 friends were deemed 'too skinny and pale'. I felt accepted and part of the normal population.

The UK was then only beginning on the path towards the epidemic of obesity. I guess I could claim to be one of the pioneers of the trend but it isn't a claim that I desire.

As an overweight student nurse who had difficulty in obtaining uniforms to fit, my ignorance was shameful. I 'sniffed' at stories of people having their teeth removed to have their jaws wired. I joined others in 'tutt-tutting' when people had lengthy open operations simply to lose weight. Key-hole surgery was simply not around in the 1970's.

Fat people were, at times, deemed to be selfish, often ignorant and a nuisance, as they were difficult to care for and less able to move following open surgery.

Sadly, death was not unknown following such operations and long term complications, including kidney failure was also later recognised as a complication of this early weight loss surgery.

The 1980's brought more globalisation and growing sizes. Special retail outlets appeared for the 'larger clientele' and well known stores 'went up to' a size that was said quietly.

"Do you sell wedding dresses big enough for my daughter?" I could almost touch the embarrassment my mother felt having a 'fat daughter bride'. I felt my own humiliation when it was reported to my father that, surprisingly, we had managed to buy a wedding dress 'big enough'.

For me the 1980's and 90's brought me; slimming tablets of varying types, weight loss, weight gain, weight loss and even more gain. As my size increased so too did my growing physical inability in simple everyday things. I was breathlessness after a short walk, tired and developed postnatal depression. I was not able to run with my children, hold a child on my lap, because I simply didn't have a lap!

I was desperate to play the guitar but couldn't see the strings when I held it.

I remember feeling utterly panic stricken .... where would I buy clothes once I couldn't buy them on the high street anymore? I was a size 30 /32 and no escape.

To lose a few pounds was easy but to lose half my body weight was impossible.

Death and a new beginning

My father died suddenly in 2000. I realised, as do many of us when we lose a parent, that he wasn't immortal.

If he wasn't immortal then that meant no one else was, including me.

I had tried everything in an attempt to change shape and size.

My flame for life was flickering and so many times I wished that it would blow out.

Serendipity and my introduction to gastric banding.

I realise now that serendipity is a 'funny old thing'.

Only a few houses away from my home lived an ex patient whose babies I had delivered. So near and yet we had not seen each other for years. When we met again she was far from the vibrant slim attractive woman I had known. Although well presented and beautifully made up she looked so old and at least 7 sizes bigger than I remembered her.

She was desperate and, as she crossed the road to talk to me, neither of us realised where this conversation would lead.

We spoke the same language and had the same desperation and a deep understanding of what we felt was our inescapable incarceration.

'I'm going to France to have a band'. I had no idea what she was talking about and her explanation was far from scientific. She was, in my mind, clearly more than slightly 'off her trolley'!

I fell into my 'well rehearsed', scripted behaviours, thoughts and feelings. Clearly she lacked any self control. How ridiculous to have an operation to lose weight. Could she just not stop eating and exercise more?

Three months later I was catching the plane and beginning my own journey from the same hospital.

I had surgery in 2000. I estimate that at the time I was one of approximately 20 people in the UK who chose to travel to Lyon to have surgery with Vincent Frering.

The UK had not fallen behind in developing bariatric services, it was, quite simply relatively unheard of and only performed by about 5 surgeons who had, I suggest, vision for change.Only those few years ago to 'need' surgery was then deemed shameful, irresponsible and even selfish. Clearly someone who 'needed' to resort to surgery lacked self control and was already often deemed a social outcast.

My life light was flickering.

I rationalised that I would die with or without the band but perhaps my life light would shine longer with the band.

My journey had begun ....

Chapter 2

SHANGRI-LA

Being fat & Shangri-La

Shangri-La, the myth of an earthly lost paradise. Perhaps this is, to some degree, what I sought with my food relationship and my body shape and size. What a wonderful place this could be for a size 32 woman who used food to give all that a magical place may offer.

A lost paradise, this magical story of Shangri-La is one of the most enduring and endearing in the world.

Shangri-La, a story that has been evident in many cultures for many thousands of years, in one form or another. The appeal for so many of us, including me, is that it is an escape, a magical positive existence. Even now, once again, I feel myself drawn to this comfortable dream like place as I type.

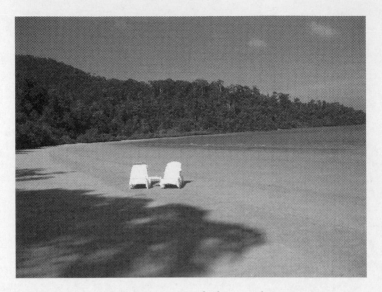

Shangri-La – a safe, happy place

I recognise how much I desired to be held in such a safe space and how I used food in an attempt to experience a little of my understanding of my own Shangri-La. Peace, acceptance, comfort, joy, solace, love, safety and pleasure. Such basic emotions seemingly fulfilled by food and eating behaviours.

For us all life has rough and tumble experiences and being very fat brings with it it's own unique problems. Shangri-La offers a dream, a possible escape from problem solving, decision making and consistency as opposed to inconsistency. I guess something we may all yearn for at stages in our lives.

Imagine, in rough times, that we could escape from our

reality, live in harmony with the world and nature, hold still the ravages of time on our body knowing that this dream like place would be where only positivity was known. Wisdom, peace and gentleness would be present, protected and perfected for us and for all in Shangri-La. I imagine floating on my back in warm waters of a beautiful, slow flowing, tropical river with no dangers around simply 'being' and being part of all that surrounds me.

Yet where would food, eating and my body fit in my lost paradise?

Would it be an abundance of any food? Continual consumption of anything I so desired? No need for physical ingestion of food? I wonder, would release from the physical negativity of fatness be the most important? Would there be a 'joy' of never needing to fulfil a 'something' or an emotion through eating? Would the release from surrounding stressors mean that food fulfilled its simple role of being a fuel and a medicine?

My personal Shangri-La is likely to be very different from yours but I suspect that as a fat person I had many similarities to others.

I am aware that for many of us we want to reach that sacred place and attain release from the physical and emotional issues associated with 'being fat'.

Legs that chafe, breasts that are pendulous or an overhanging stomach, that is red raw with soreness. The dreadful experiences of excess sweating, not being able to tie your own shoe laces or being forced to buy in a select number of shops is only part of what we so want to be released from.

We can become so used to not succeeding. How easy it can be to plug into our 'dark side', the negative side, of our character and focus on and personalise our failings. Our personal windows of choice are sealed and the steel blinds pulled down to banish any positive light, logic or sound.

Readily blaming our 'self' for being and then in an attempt to 'improve' we try to live by pre-scripted or 'fixed' rules of restriction and admonishment if we stray. Falling ever more deeply into despondency and lack of self belief when we have a 'scale number disaster' we then stray from the straight unrealistic rules we have laid down for ourselves. To outsiders it can seem a ridiculous situation a mountain from tiny mole hill simply by gaining 2lbs in a day. To us it is not.

For many of us, who have been locked into the diet cycle, huge value is given to rules and expectations that may have been laid down for years. Often from a now 'dated' diet book or a faded photograph of when we were fleetingly a size 12 achieved by a, 'water and cracker only' intake for weeks.

Being overly concerned about what 'ought', 'should' or 'must be' blinds us from acceptance, clear thought and the ability to hear and our fear and catastrophisation is allowed to rule our personal roost.

These are all complex factors and somehow, in my view, these issues can dull our vision of what may be involved in the creation and maintenance of remaining fat for whatever reason. Even if you have weight loss surgery these can be issues that will need to be addressed.

How does 'being fat' serve you?

When I ask patients this question it is often met with utter disbelief and the indignant retort of, 'it doesn't'!

So, why, if it doesn't serve us do we choose to remain fat?

Some people have a gentle realisation and will say – 'ahh yes it does serve me, it means that x will bring me food, do xyz for me and I am cared for'.

If I was thin I'd have to do this myself on my own" …. Of course some realise that their 'significant other' is party to, or in collusion with, the game of 'keep X fat' as it enables maintaining familiar feelings of 'abc' which is a safe place to be fixed in.

One lady, who is bed bound, shared with me that for her it means her 13 year old daughter comes to tend to her and feed her and show her love. It means more to her to remain the same than risk losing this special time and relationship she values with her daughter.

For some it is simply protective to have a cushion of adipose wrapped around them feels safe. It may repel the opposite sex, it may be simply comfortable.

Being fat did serve me in many peculiar ways, some at an emotional level and some at a physical level. In many ways being fat 'drove' me. I had to prove I could do better, work harder, be happier, be most liked and be the most able even though I was the biggest member of staff.

For many of us a time may come when we need professional help in exploring associated emotions, behaviours and thoughts.

Some of us need to ask ourselves about what is keeping us where we are?

Do we want to change, is it worth the risk? Can we walk into the unknown and risk being in a shape and size that may be totally unknown to us? Would our significant others reject us or sabotage us?

Weight loss, change of shape and size does not come without personal cost.

Many people lose friends when they are no longer 'the bet at the end of the bar' or the 'token fat friend'. When you become attractive to others you may become a threat and, sadly, couples do part. As shape and size change so too do the people involved.

It was difficult for my daughters to see me beginning to value my new body, putting make-up on, choosing new clothes and not inevitably standing in front of the cooker whipping up wonderful comfort foods. Mummy changed and it wasn't always comfortable to see someone who they didn't know move in instead.

Sometimes, being challenged gently by a professional can be helpful. To be asked what evidence there is to sustain some of the thoughts that contribute to remaining the same. For some of us it may be helpful to unpick some of the related food and eating behaviours.

On the other hand some prefer to let sleeping dogs lie and move on to behavioural change and weight loss surgery without questioning.

Personal reflection

I said goodbye to a good friend that was leaving my department this week. We met a couple of years ago initially as work colleagues and this had developed to a friendship that whenever I felt emotional highs or lows it was to her office that I migrated. We shared our feelings together either over a cup of coffee (we were at work after all) and chocolate biscuit or with yet another box of tissues to mop up the tears and the running mascara.

When she left I asked her to keep in touch and made sure that both of us were armed with every conceivable means of doing so. Various phone numbers and e-mail addresses were exchanged and filed away in the crevices of our purses but even before I said the final farewell, I knew that mine would never come out and see the light of day.

Not because I didn't want to or because I didn't mean what I had just said about keeping in touch but because I could not accept that she wanted to know me. How could she possibly want to know the ugly fat woman who sat alone in the corner?

There was my friend, a very successful woman at the peak of her career, happily married, very attractive, size eight and a great personality and there was me, fat, ugly and an emotional failure. How could she possibly want to ever talk to me or arrange to meet for lunch and be seen with me?

I then started to think of how relationships change because of the feeling of lack of self worth and with it came the realisation that body size and the lowering of self esteem crept into so many aspects of our lives. By keeping in contact with someone would then lay me open to the possibility of rejection so it became easier to severe the relationship and crawl back into the corner on my own, rather than face that possibility.

The anticipation of rejection becomes part of life and so easy to put down to body size and image. It is easier to make sure that the rejection cannot happen and hurt us so we turn our backs on life and the company of others and make sure that no one gets close enough.

It starts at a young age.

The choosing of the teams at school with the teacher selecting ' Miss blonde and beautiful' and 'Miss perfectly proportioned with legs up to her armpits' as the team captains. They alternately select the girls to join them, all clones of the captains and all as equally as gorgeous but then it gets harder as it gets down to the remaining unselected two girls. The fat, useless one and the one that doesn't participate in team activities as she is too busy reading Plato. I never got selected and no, I don't read Plato.

Then there is the day when the teacher has the bright idea of making those two girls the team captains to avoid their embarrassment of always being selected last. This solves nothing as 'Miss blonde and beautiful' and 'Miss perfectly proportioned' are forced reluctantly towards their teams so the rejection is still there just packaged differently.

As the years pass comes the annual, ultimate rejection and humiliation. Valentine's Day. As all the beautiful girls are counting and comparing the size of cards (and believe me when it comes to valentine cards, size does matter) that are declaring undying passionate love from an anonymous admirer it becomes easier to post a card to yourself to avoid the rejection from this exclusive club. It is also worth it to see the look of disbelief on the other girls' faces when the fat girl can also have tangible proof of being physically attractive to the opposite sex.

Later in life, Valentine cards, or the lack of them, can be explained away by the late arrival of the postman and fortunately by February 15th no one seems to care how many cards were received.

The next rejection comes with the nights out with girl friends to parties and night clubs. All the other girls are dressed in the last outfit from the latest designer who caters for size six to ten. Skin tight jeans that look moulded to the wearers legs, knee high black boots and the skimpiest, floaty, delicate top that just about covers her ample cleavage. And then there is the fat girl. The extra large black, loose trousers and the black top that covers everything from neck to thighs. It has to be black as darker colours not only make fat people look thinner but it enables them to blend into the background of a dark dance floor so that no one notices that they are dancing alone. Everyone is reassuring that you look good but you know that they are only being kind and that they need you to go along to look after them when Romeo gets too over powering or when they have had too much to drink and they need someone to stand outside the toilet door.

Then there is the humiliation of being the only person that is never asked to dance. After all some one has to be left at the table to look after the drinks. So when all the other girls in the group are having a good time on the dance floor in the arms of their latest conquest the fat girl is left looking on pretending it doesn't matter and they don't care. So the feeling of rejection and being singled out continues. When the prayers for the floor to open up are unanswered it is easier to leave everyone else having a good time and go home to the ever loving plate of chips and mayo that never offers rejection.

And so the cycle continues. What initially started as rejection of the fat child and the fat adolescent stays with us through life and shapes our relationships with others that we meet along the way.

The thought that they may want to know me for what I am and that my size is totally irrelevant never crosses my mind. It is totally beyond my comprehension as I only see the fat, ugly person that stands in front of me in the mirror.

So, will these feelings ever go away? As the pounds (I pray) gradually peel away will the ingrained emotions peel away with it? How can a lifetime of ensuring that others do not see the hurt and rejection be changed? The simple....... I don't know.

The one thing I do know is that it will not put me off from trying and if I still see myself as the ugly, somewhat thinner person in the corner then that is something I will have to deal with and face at a later date.

I'm not worth it.....

Weight loss surgery is an external event it does not become who I am and I do not become 'weight loss surgery'. How many of us have seen the card that says –

"Wine is made to be drunk. I am drunk therefore, am I wine???"

As fat people, we are highly geared to food as a reward or as a comfort. We use food as a method of communicating both outwardly and inwardly. We can express love by feeding those close to us and feeding ourselves. We can soothe ourselves, anaesthetise our hurts and nurture ourselves.

Where are we? Have we had our sense of autonomy miscoded by continual dieting and reliance on numbers, weights or restrictive rules and regulations?

How can we develop or restore a sense of our own autonomy? Have we ever lived a self sufficient life or always been dependant on relationship with others or food?

What did life feel like then or, what does it feel like considering becoming an independent adult? Is there something that is likely to hold us or destroy us from achieving a sense of self sufficiency? How does what, when, and why we eat fit in to this?

Weight loss surgery – whatever type is only a tool, a vehicle to enable our physical self to become smaller. We cannot rely 100% on a surgical procedure to change our body, mind and spirit. We have to change in the understanding of ourselves and continually walk the walk of understanding, new knowledge and behavioural changes. It is not all about weight and weight loss and success need not be measured by numbers on the scale alone.

It is well known that people don't change or do things 'because it's good for them' or because their current situation is hurting.

These may motivate an approach to change but it is a complex intertwining of processes that is involved. I know I would benefit from increasing my activity I am motivated to do so however I chose, at this time, not to because I feel more comfortable as I am.

Psychological research indicates that fat people tend to judge and be very judgemental of their own behaviour. Basically, you are likely to be very hard on yourself!

Part of the process is the introduction of possible new ideas of how can you take care of you and value you?

Interestingly, there is a suggestion that many fat people have developed poor problem solving skills. This, in turn, leads to being safe in our avoidance and denial that we have any size related issues. We are also deemed to be impulsive in behaviour and that impulsivity may be triggered by various stimulants – smell, taste, venue, emotion. Can you smell popcorn by the way?

Social v Physical

Whatever social connotations that are assumed about fat people I feel that it is rarely acknowledged that it is, quite simply, hard work being fat.

It is physically hard work and very tiring to move and manoeuvre a heavy object on a daily basis. It can be even harder when so much of the time we attempt to appear 'normal', even agile, to 'prove' we are able.

It is hard work to maintain personal hygiene – 'just in case'. I remember trying to fit a shower into my schedule several times each summer day because, 'I may smell'.

Socially, yes fat people may be deemed to be happy or the 'life and soul'. Many carrying a heavy and huge, 'mask of happiness' to distract from the appearing shape and size. Of course I'm not saying all fat people are like this, or that all fat people are miserable. Simply over time it appears that 'jolly happy' people are often portrayed as being fat.

Yet there is a strange dichotomy. How many time have I either felt, or had said to me by a patient, 'people think I am stupid, greedy, lazy and all I do is sit round all day watching soaps on TV and eating'. I frequently meet clients who have these 'mindreading assumptions' – but are they assumptions?

The 'but you've got such a pretty face' comment wears a bit thin when your heading out of one XL size into an

XXL size and you have been asked by a three year old if you have a baby in your tummy for the second time in a week.

Fat people are sadly evaluated by shape and size. Many people I see have formed an outer shell to support this objective evaluation to the point that some do not recognise the whole self. The essence and core strength of who they are as an individual, a unique and special person. A finely tuned, delicate and sensitive creation the whole 'self' that contributes to sustaining our physical shape and size.

Often people arrive to first consultation troubled, some fearful of judgement and retribution. They leave, I hope with positive affirmation and non judgemental acceptance that they have a chronic disease.

I could count on one hand clients who have come through our service who have a significant psychiatric illness. Yet, historically fat people have been deemed mentally ill or even 'mad' (whatever that term actually means).

Somehow it remains socially acceptable to say 'I'm on a diet' – indeed one almost 'becomes acceptable'. However it seems less acceptable to say 'I'm frightened, I need help, I've tried everything and now I would like to consider weight loss surgery'.

The people I meet are, in the main, wanting to take control of an area of their lives that, to date, they have not been able to. Is someone who is seeking a surgical intervention to help reduce body size any more or any less emotionally 'toxic' than someone who doesn't chose this route? I don't believe so.

Assessment

At the initial assessment, I ask the person many questions but one is – why are you seeking surgery?

I suspect one word, 'desperation', would cover much of what is said but somewhere it includes, 'I have tried everything, nothing works… I have no willpower or self control'. Yet these are the very people who have possibly starved themselves on ridiculously low calorie diets for weeks, 'eaten' only liquid for months (or longer), have stuck to cabbage soup, grapefruit or other interesting combinations in hope of reaching the mystical Shangri-La of 'slim'. The direction on the 'diet map of hopefulness', is being given and directed by an outsider. Usually it is heavily based on restriction and judgemental outcomes more often based on reduction of numbers.

Coercion – 'go on a diet' can activate negative reactions and the opposite effect may happen. What happens when we 'finish' (which is a challenging term alone) a regime of unnatural eating?

Our bodies seek nutrition and fuel. Quite naturally the body seeks food. To eat normal food again is, of course, natural and the experience of pleasure and satisfaction is also normal. Food is a substance designed to satisfy. It is a fuel and, I have to agree with those who say, a medicine also.

To listen to our bodies and hear our bodies needs in seeking fuel and medicine does not mean that we have 'failed' or 'lapsed'. We simply require to eat and then for possible scripted reasons then beat ourselves up for stepping outside the straight lines of 'ridiculous restriction rules' that we believe to be 'the' way.

Perhaps a medal not self flagellation would be the more appropriate outcome?! Well done for listening and hearing that your body seeks nutrition. Now chose wisely and eat mindfully.

So much of this is not broached when surgery to aid weight loss is explored and yet so much of this, in my opinion, is vital to increase our understanding and hopefully change in shape and size – to whatever that we chose it to be.

Hopefully, following weight loss surgery, a gradual outward physical change will happen. Yet for many the physical change is only part of the total picture. Change of job, challenges in partnership, grief process and increased self belief are common following weight loss. I believe we can learn to value more than weight loss itself. We can value change and even more simply we can learn to value who we are over and above what our size and shape is.

Weight loss is the cherry on the cake. The cake and the white icing are the behavioural and life style changes that the journey involves and it takes time.

Medical advantage to losing weight.

I cannot think of many fat people who don't know that there are medical advantages of being a smaller shape and size.

After all, we are the ones who wake in the night because we have to 'turn' our bodies in bed. In the morning we promise, once again, to 'try' because of our health, children, longevity, illness etc until the words become meaningless as the resulting emotions are dulled with our food related actions.

Most of us know that weight loss has been recognised for many years to have a significant, positive impact and improvement both on many diseases and also, therefore, prolonged life expectancy.

I think it is important to realise that obesity is a chronic disease. Much like any other it simply doesn't 'go away' or diminish. Indeed, the incidence of obesity is growing in most industrialised countries and the impact at a socioeconomic level is also growing in significance.

The 'too fat to work' scenario is now recognised and the financial impact of obesity on health systems is said to be the second most expensive of all chronic diseases in the

USA and parts of Europe. (The World Health organisation) - http://www.who.int/mediacentre/factsheets/fs311/en/index.html)

Abdominal obesity, the classic 'beer belly' and the increased risk of heart disease is now well known as, 'The metabolic syndrome'.

Medical terminology can be somewhat 'mind boggling' and unpronounceable but increasingly we hear or read terms such as: Insulin Resistance, Raised fasting glucose, hyperinsulineamia, type two diabetes, dyslipideamia, hyperlipdeamia, raised cholesterol and high blood pressure.

When you see the word 'syndrome' it means a collection of symptoms or recognised features. Even more simply put, our bodies are struggling because of the volume of food we eat, the quality of foods and therefore chemicals we chose to eat and the types of fluid we choose to consume, usually in excess.

It is said that Obesity is to become the 'norm' in many states of the USA within only a couple of years. When one considers the volume, frequency and food types consumed it never ceases to amaze me that someone can consume such quantities.

Clearly it is more logical to treat the cause of a problem that the symptoms.

I could easily keep a bowl under a dripping pipe and regularly empty it however it seems far more logical to mend the fault in the pipe, or replace the pipe.

There is little difference with illnesses. It is well known that weight loss forms part of the treatment to improve metabolic syndrome by treating the cause i.e. being fat.

Health benefits

Even a 5% or 10 % loss of weight can lead to significant improvement of such things as diabetes.

Saying goodbye to 10kgs of fat is said to :

- Decrease death rate by 20-25%
- Decrease Diabetes related deaths by 30-40%
- Decrease Obesity-related cancer deaths 40-50%.
- Lower Blood pressure
- Reduce the symptoms of high blood pressure up to 90%
- Increases the ability to move and increase activity
- Cholesterol lowered.
- Decrease the risk of developing diabetes by more than 50%

I am amazed that such a small weight loss can have such a huge positive potential impact. Even for those who have none of the above conditions it is significant in not developing them.

I guess many of us know these facts but are able to dissociate from them. It won't happen to me and actually they are, 'only words'.

Someone came to see me today. I asked her, 'How did you feel when you were told that you had Type 2 diabetes?'

Her answer, 'Nothing, because I knew it was likely to happen the fatter I got. Now I've got it I don't want the illnesses it brings and I want to keep my sight and I don't want those leg ulcers they get'.

The inevitable has arrived for this lady and, as prepared as she was to be diagnosed with such a silent and destructive disease she chose to continue to feed her emotional needs using food and she now wants to unpick what she has created and sustained.

We can explore personal therapy, alternative therapies, prescribed medication, surgery, activity increase but, at the end of the day – quite annoyingly but totally logically - it always boils down to how much we put into our mouths is too much!

To work out how to understand what, how, when and where of eating often means we need some professional, non-judgemental insight that may come in many different forms.

Personally, I loathe the title 'dietician'. It has too many personal historical connotations for me. Thankfully, in the 45 + years since I first met with a dietician they have changed. Certainly, the ones I know have skilled insight in helping the development of eating related behavioural change. The ones I know do not 'buy into' admonishment but explore how to introduce change.

Long term, for some, it is very difficult to sustain such change simply with modification of lifestyle without support. For this group medical or surgical intervention is an additional tool that may be considered.

Weight loss surgery in recent years has been proclaimed the most successful in sustaining excess weight loss. For many this is sold as a miracle, the 'wonder surgery' something that is permanent.

Not a miracle cure

The truth …. no surgery performed for management of weight is guaranteed and none is the simple answer for sustained loss.

Many people gain weight after 3-5 years be that with more interventionist procedures – e.g. gastric bypass or surgery that is deemed the 'safest' i.e. gastric banding.

I have a few friends who have had what I heard once deemed the 'platinum' weight loss surgery procedure – The Duodenal Switch. Both have sadly gained weight and both now have numerous physical and psychological issues still unresolved.

With an operation may come new complications.

It is for this reason that I feel anyone considering weight loss surgery should research and really understand not only the 'procedure' but also what to expect. It is not about reaching a pot of gold at the base of the rainbow. It is about understanding that you are buying into a life style change for life.

I work with wonderful surgeons who I respect hugely. They are highly skilled and experienced professionals who I would certainly trust with my life.

No matter how skilled and how experienced they are unlikely to instigate our personal behavioural change. They can contribute to giving us the best possible help but it is 'down to us' to accept the responsibility of being an adult in all areas of our lives. Only we can live our life and walk our walk.

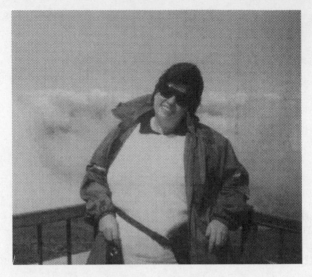

Me on top of Mount Washington 1998.
6,288 feet above mean sea level

Chapter 3

PREPARING FOR SURGERY

Is this really for me?

So you want to make some changes? Remember this is for life. Much as parenthood or similar commitments, remember this too is 'not just for Christmas'.

Can you introduce some early changes before you go any further with your journey?

Before you go to your GP, ask yourself some penetrating questions. No one but you will be living with your weight loss surgery and the resulting journey, be that a happy one, or an unhappy one.

I can assure you, if you chose to go ahead it will take

physical and psychological energy and is no way to be considered the 'easy way out'.

How am I when dealing or introducing change into my life?

You may know that you need to reduce your shape and size and be very willing to do so. Remember that change is an active process. You have to be committed to take part in an active process and this active process depends on your willingness to work with you and the necessary changes.

Is this the time I am going to put aside to give to ME?

Let's face it if you are planning a wedding, having a baby, worried about work or money or have had a recent loss or bereavement this takes up huge emotional space.

Is this really the best time to introduce something else to contend with? Having surgery won't take any of the above away it will simply add to them.

It doesn't mean never but maybe it could mean, 'in a while' when you are able to concentrate 100% on you. We are all capable of overloading our ability and set ourselves up for less success with poor planning.

I want to wake up tomorrow and be thin - can I cope with reality?

One of the most common things with us all is that we want to go to bed and wake up slender, or very slender.

I have yet to work out where all the adipose would have been when I woke, or indeed what clothes I would have been able to wear had this miracle happened.

It would form part of my dream world but I am not sure if I could have coped had it happened.

Somehow we forget how long it has taken to get to the shape and size we are and how long it takes to reverse it.

It is likely to take between 18 months and 2 years to get to the shape and size you feel at peace with. Slow weight loss is safer and is easier to maintain. Rapid weight loss may mean muscle loss. Muscle burns calories at a high rate and ... there are many muscles in your body, including your heart muscle.

Who around me would prefer me to stay the size I am?

Are they likely to sabotage your efforts because it is better for them if you don't change?

That's a tough point as it includes who you may see as current friends and is highly possible to include close family.

Belief.

I know that you can do this!

I have never met you but I know by reaching out for this book you are in the right mindset to consider this as an option.

I equally know that if everything is in place and you are willing, ready and able to change that you will succeed.

Behavioural change

I was very angry tonight I ate and ate as much as I could, until I hurt.

My anger is still there and so are about 3,000 extra calories.

All this sounds so easy in theory but when you hit the wall of emotion are you willing to learn enough to be able to choose and understand that you can challenge your established copy behaviours?

Sounds easy to do in theory, but in practice, it is difficult.

Activity

Please, please, please don't immediately rush to your local gym or book in for the 'Bath Half Marathon'!

Start with the simple question, 'how can I increase my **A**ctivity?'. Note it is the 'A' word and not the 'E' word (exercise!).

Start simply, do things that some take for granted. Can you hang the washing out on the line or take the pile of ironing from the bottom of the stairs up to the top of the stairs?

These seem small changes to introduce but such seemingly small tasks can be such exhausting mountains to climb when you are much bigger than you would like to be.

If you are really desperate to 'do' the 'E' word then look at Yoga, Pilates, Aqua-robics and seek professional help in managing such exercise. They will understand the body's mechanics and how the muscles and ligaments work for those who are not used to exercise and those who are larger than many.

Go gently because to go back to the introduction being fat is hard work.

It is harder work to do some seemingly simply everyday jobs when you are already carrying an extra load.

Change

Changing any established behaviour isn't easy.

For some time my family, now composed of 4 adults, have

only to walk a few extra paces to put the recycling waste into one container to be taken to a local recycling centre. Recently, the frequency and manner in which recycling is to be stored and collected has changed.

Oh my goodness, the confusion! New colours, new bins, increased frequency of collection, change of days and some weekly to fortnightly collections have introduced new 'challenges' to my family.

The major overhaul of understanding and what they need to change has been somewhat interesting to say the least!

They have now to walk the extra paces and think before they dispose. They have had to think and recognise what we have been doing and now what we need to do.

It takes time and effort and no wonder that the local authority started the process of introducing change some 4 months in advance!

Change can be introduced slowly and begun with easy things first. No one expects you to have a behavioural 'make-over' over night. You may still choose to hold on to some of those things that you feel comfortable with, or ones that you don't want to change. The key is to start your change slowly and simply.

When I lay in bed in the morning, trying hard to cling to those vital few minutes extra of relaxation, I would listen to my husband getting ready for work.

His routine became fascinating for me when I was learning about change. I feel certain that his routine was totally unrecognised and unknown to him, until he reads this.

Each weekday morning, he would get ready in the same way. Having dressed and eaten breakfast he would track his shoes down. I knew his process would finish by him returning to our bedroom, going to the top drawer, taking out his hair brush and brushing his hair with eight strokes. How do I know – because I counted them regularly.

To introduce change for my husband may mean to simply brush his hair at the beginning of his daily pattern or with a few extra brush strokes.

This simple introduction of change would then contribute to change his learnt pattern and perhaps make him more aware of surroundings and actions.

What could you do to change your routines? Put your right shoe on instead of your left? Change your mascara colour? Throw your toothbrush away and break out for a different colour. All these small things start to move us away from what, so easily, become fixed habits.

Yep, you will battle it because we like comfort zones, we like easy non challenging lives but you are contemplating one of the biggest life-long changes of your life so start thinking before you move to the next step.

Chapter 4

GETTING THE BALL ROLLING...

Approaching professionals.

This is a guide on the processes and pitfalls on taking weight loss beyond the diet books to the next level. It highlights the options and the best ways of approaching professionals. It touches on the medical and the surgical options (of which there are many) available to the patient. Once referral has been accepted, this guides the patient right up to the operating room door.

How to approach your GP

Patient story .....

I was told I had high blood pressure and my GP told me to go away and lose weight. No help to how I was going to achieve this. By this time I had already explored all the slimming clubs, done the Woman's Weekly 'lose a dress size in two weeks' and knew the calorific value of every ready meal in Tesco. The enormity of being told to go away and lose weight was too much. In so many ways my GP was extremely supportive and understanding but as she was a size 10 herself she obviously had no idea of what she was asking. Each time I went back to have my blood pressure checked I was a nervous wreck anticipating how long into my appointment the subject of how much I had lost would be. No wonder my blood pressure was always high. If she did not say anything I would breathe a sigh of relief as I walked out of the surgery and thinking thank goodness I had got away with it although I knew I would not be so lucky at the next visit.

How many other people that are floundering in an abyss of despair concerning their health and weight continue to stay there because they cannot ask a professional medically trained person for help? Equally why do GP's not realise that the overweight patient sitting in front of them does not choose to ignore their warnings of the consequences of be overweight but cannot do it alone and without an enormous amount of support?

Probably if I had had the confidence to tell my doctor all this and could put into words how I felt she would have offered support but for most overweight people the ability to verbalise their feelings is not an option. It takes a lot of bravery to finally admit that help is required and even then the feelings of guilt and lack of self worth prevents all aspects from being discussed.

If someone presented with lung cancer that had smoked 50 days for all their adult life and still continued to smoke after diagnosis then most people would turn on them and say 'what did they expect' and should the NHS be wasting precious resources in treating them when their condition was self afflicted.

Similar logic surrounds someone who is overweight.

It is my fault that I am this size. No one forced me to eat. My addiction to food I realise now was for many reasons but all of which resulted in me putting food into my mouth. Therefore I am responsible for my size in the same way as the person who smoked 50 a day so have I the right to go and ask for help.

Take courage

If you have tried every diet known to mankind and have also tried prescribed medication then, what have you got to you lose?

You are likely to have memorised all the red and green foods, know the points in a carrot and may even have gone the 'ketosis' way. In reality, you are likely to know the ins and outs of most vogue diets. What fat content is in 25gms of cheese and how much hoovering you need to do before rewarding yourself with another chocolate digestive.

Your book shelves are bulging with booklets that have semi completed personal weight graphs in the back and curled pages where you have religiously followed weird and wonderful menus that are 'cure-alls' to this condition of obesity, if only.

Little wonder you are desperate, exhausted and are willing to grasp at a passing lettuce leaf for help. This ghastly place is only too familiar and you don't want to be there anymore.

For some of us we have to 'steel ourselves' before we pick up the phone to make the appointment. I recognise only too well that it's a brave soul who can walk into the GP and say 'I've had enough', 'I'm too fat and I need help' ... pleeeeeeeeeeease help me.

Some of us know only too well that our Dr will decide that weight loss is a novel cure for a 'verruca'. You know the type? ....*Well Sharon, if you could only lose some weight 'it' would be better* - whatever the presenting 'it' of the moment is at that time.

The well practiced, "Eat less and do more exercise" type of consultation really does not help someone who has tried, tried, tried and tried again and not succeeded. We know how to emotionally 'barricade ourselves' or hold the happy & reasonable 'mask of protection' in front of our faces, as that old chestnut is voiced from the other side of a desk.

I guess I would love to have been rescued by the 'Dr with the magic wand'. That would have meant I could sit back and simply let it 'happen' as he waived his magic 'Dr wand' and 'whoosh' all was slender.

What we really want is a road map. We don't need to be rescued but do need to be to be heard and valued. No one can 'do' this for us. However, to be accepted and recognised as someone 'worthwhile' would be good.

I had one client who was asked by their GP, did they know how to loose 10kgs of ugly fat? The client, so pleased at possible helpful input, answered "no, how"? His GP answered .."Chop your head off"!

Little wonder that many of us are reticent to seek help. Guess what though, it is not necessarily going to be a 'tough call'. As time has gone on more awareness and training has been given to the subject of 'obesity' and Dr's seem to be developing a healthier understanding and becoming more approachable to the idea of weight loss surgery as an option.

Let me say that again – it may not be as bad as you expect and may be even better than you expect!

Plan your consultation

Did you realise that GP's are given very little time to spend with us – usually 10 minutes? In this time they are expected to see, diagnose and sort what are often very complicated cases. So PLAN what to say and how you will say it.

Some people find it very helpful to write a letter to their GP before the appointment so that the ground is prepared. Some find it useful to take a list of points for the appointment.

You are human you may get nervous, gabble your words or even 'bottle out' when you get face to face so please PLAN ahead.

You may think that to include some of the following may be useful:-

- Obviously I get very upset about such a personal issue as my shape and size and that is why I have written this letter before I see you. I would like to discuss the option of weight loss surgery with you.

- As you know I have been a patient with you for X yrs.

- I have tried, as you know, xyz methods to lose weight and maintain the loss but to date have been unsuccessful.

- I am getting to the point physically that I know I have to lose weight. I am no longer able to..

  ○ tie my laces,

- ◦ go shopping alone (or at all),

- ◦ put on my tights,

- ◦ get clothes to fit,

- ◦ tend to my personal hygiene,

- ◦ walk more than x paces etc

- As you know I have now developed conditions that I understand are liked to being overweight e.g.

  - ◦ I am type 2 diabetic

  - ◦ My asthma has worsened

  - ◦ My blood pressure has increased

  - ◦ I am more depressed

  - ◦ etc etc

- I have researched various types of weight loss and understand the different options as I understand them to be.

- I have been to a local support group / have spoken to other people who have had weight loss surgery. Give your GP the details of this group.

- I have asked about positive and negative aspects and although I am obviously apprehensive remaining the same is too difficult a situation and not one I want to stay in.

- I would be grateful if you could refer me to a team who specialise in weight management and who have long term experience in weight loss surgery and the management.

How supportive are GPs to weight loss?

GP's are in the unusual position of needing to know a great deal about a number of conditions. As with hospital doctors, they may have a greater interest in specialities that do not include surgery. Some, however, may have wondered if they should go down the surgery training route and therefore have a greater interest. As with all individuals they may, sadly, have preconceived ideas of what constitutes a 'fat person' or what weight loss surgery means.

You will be seeking support and advice in an area s/he may know little about so approach with an open mind and be clear in what you are seeking.

What is their reaction to weight loss surgery?

Again, this depends on their knowledge, experience and/ or lack of both. It may be likely that older GP's remember the early weight loss procedures that had a high death rate associated to them and to those who had long term complications with their kidneys or other organs. Perhaps your GP has very strong views and is very 'fattist' or even anti surgery?

However, your GP may be very pleased that you mentioned

it as s/he had been waiting for the 'right moment' to suggest it to you!

Plan your reactions for any eventuality and above all try to hear her/his side as well as your own. Most GP's genuinely want to give a balanced view and appreciate many of the aspects of your life that you may not realise.

You won't know until you have that appointment and, who knows, you may be pleasantly surprised.

At what stage do GPs refer patients?

I was told by an NHS manager many years ago,

"Sharon you care too much. This is a service lead industry"

Sadly this, in many ways, has continued.

Less often is a GP able to be a 'Dr Finlay' type knowing the family for years and understanding the complexities of the family. Your GP is faced with a delicate balanced of time, professionalism and keeping their housekeeping money in order.

GP's, as other health practitioners are directed to 'follow a pathway' or recommended practice and this will impact on what happens next. They have to tick the boxes laid down by parties such as NICE or the Department of Health. While you may think it is ridiculous (they too may feel this way) it simply is part of 'the system' that you will find yourself in.

So please expect to be somewhat touched or affected by the system you are entering.

You are likely to be 'categorised' (see BMI below), you may possibly be 'herded' into tiers of weight management care, or levels of care (see below) before even a glimmer of an operation is visible. So please, if you are walking the NHS route, be prepared for several detours to get to your goal.

In the UK the government established 'National Institute for Health and Clinical Excellence' (NICE) and describe themselves as

" *.. an independent organisation responsible for providing national guidance on promoting good health and preventing and treating ill health* ". http://www.nice.org.uk/

This organisation recommend that weight loss surgery is available as a treatment option for those people who are morbidly or 'super' obese.

Personally, I loathe the terminology 'morbidly obese' but I have to say it was the ONLY time in my life I was glad to be that ghastly term *'morbidly obese'* !

I prefer to say thank goodness I was 'fat enough'!

BODY MASS INDEX

Body Mass Index was invented by Adolphe Quetelet, a Belgian Polymath, between the years 1830 and 1850. It is increasingly clear that while a BMI calculation may be useful it is somewhat limited. It doesn't, for example, demonstrate distribution of body fat or where fat may be stored.

To find out if you are 'Morbidly or super obese' you need to work out your Body Mass Index [BMI]. It is the measurement used to work out 'how fat', or not, we are! Incidentally there are growing bodies who do not think this is the most efficient way of working out our 'fatness'. Many prefer to use waist circumference however, we are stuck with this as the current recognised measure!

In scientific 'lingo':-

BMI is the ratio of a person's weight to the square of their height (both in metric units).There are many online sites that provide easy BMI calculators including mine at www. gastricbandservice.co.uk or www.avonobesityservice. co.uk

When you have worked out what your BMI is then you can be 'categorised' or slotted into a 'category'.

A BMI below 19.5 is considered underweight

- 19.5 - 25 = 'normal/desirable'

- 25 - 30 = overweight
- 30 - 40 = obese
- More than 40, or over 35 and you have weight-related problems, is classified as 'morbidly obese'.

I tend to 'balk' at being in 'a category' however, I have to put up with it as meaningless as it may be, it is a measure, a tool.

Using BMI presents a somewhat illogical situation. If one were to look at e.g. an international rugby player who is fit and has significant muscle bulk he is likely to be categorised as morbidly obese yet far from requiring surgery to aid weight loss.

Guidelines are guidelines though and, to be considered for weight loss surgery BMI is the preferred tool at this time.

It has little bearing to me on what being 'too fat' actually means. It is merely a vehicle of convenience to serve a function and distribute care, estimate financing care or aid diagnosis.

My category today, as I type this, is 'normal/desirable', I certainly don't feel either at the moment!

Yesterday one of our patients was very upset. She has lost 15stone and is very very happy as she is. She does not want to lose any more weight. She is in the 'obese' category. For her she is exactly where she wants to be. For the money holders she remains 'too fat' for a tummy tuck.

In theory, the NHS will consider you for surgery if you have scrambled up a pyramid of weight management service design = tier 1, tier 2, tier 3 and lastly tier 4. Once you have scrambled over the tiered hurdles you reach the final frontier that is set by NICE and includes :

- You are generally fit enough to have an anaesthetic and surgery
- You are aged 18 or over
- You have been receiving treatment in a weight management clinic – tier/level 3 usually at a hospital. These are medically supervised services.
- You have suffered from obesity for more than 5 years
- You have tried all other appropriate non-surgical treatments to lose weight but have not been able to maintain weight loss
- You fully understand the procedure and the need for long-term follow-up care and changing your eating habits
- You are not dependent on alcohol or drugs
- You have no untreated endocrine disorder
- There is no specific medical or psychological

reasons why weight loss surgery should not
be performed

Remember that some parts of the NHS may simply not have the money in their pot to pay for surgery. Your only other options is to pay within the private sector, as many of us have done.

Otherwise, the more familiar 'I'll try one more time because I 'should' be able to do this on my own', is likely to kick in.

I really do wish I could do, and could have done, the weight loss 'thing' without the need for surgery. I remember standing at the bottom of my mountain in awe of the enormity of my predicted journey. I had to reach the peak of losing 9stone and slipped regularly after, either a short time period, or a small weight loss.

I truly admire those who achieve it and maintain the life changes involved. I wish you could bottle whatever you have a pass it around to others!

I don't know why I couldn't do it. Perhaps I have a genuine 'missing link' somewhere, who knows. Weight loss surgery is by NO MEANS the easier option. So why have I managed with this difficult option and not without? I simply do not know.

If your GP is able to refer you to a Specialist team of professionals, either within the NHS or private sector, please expect to have an in depth consultation pre-operatively with several specialist practitioners. I consider this to be high quality practice.

Where I work for example, you would see a Physician who is a specialist in Endocrinology, Diabetes and Obesity, a Specialist Nutritionist and me (as a Specialist Nurse who is trained as a counsellor and eating disorder specialist).

Chapter 5

MEETING THE SPECIALISTS – YOU'RE NEARLY THERE!

What next?

You have made it to your GP – well done!!

You have funding from the NHS – Hurrah!!

You have decided to pay for this yourself – You ARE worth it!!

Now ... you now have the first appointment – yikes am I mad ?!?

Everywhere will differ slightly as to what happens but I will lay out what, as a practitioner, I would consider necessary if you were my mother, daughter, brother or father.

I would want the best for you from the outset and that would include knowing that you would be referred to a team of health professionals who are specifically trained in this area. You are worth more than a FIFO service i.e. 'fit it and 'fly off' service!

Hopefully, together with the research that you have already done, via word of mouth, the www, books or patient support groups you will arrive at the appointment with a tool box of information to help you and a list of questions to ask.

I would hope, and expect that, you will already have been able to ask questions on the phone, perhaps been sent some information or a questionnaire, or be given some at the initial appointment.

If you have specifics to ask - then ask them. You are likely to be paying for this make sure it is what YOU want.

These may include simple questions e.g.

- How many procedures have the team been involved with?
- What infection rate do you have?
- Have you got some patients I could speak to?
- Have you a support group I can attend?

Remember this is not a shopping trip this is about your health and you need not fear asking relevant questions that will help you decide if this is what you really want to do.

FIRST SPECIALIST CONSULTATION

What questions will you be asked at your first Specialist consultation?

Obviously you will have already passed your details on and one would expect, from a reputable team that they would have requested a letter of referral from your GP, if you are entering the private sector.

Other than that expect standard questions relating to the following:

- Social status
- Your occupation
- Your Family History
- Your Past and Current Medical conditions and history
- Your past Surgical History
- Current prescribed medication
- If you have any Allergies
- Your Smoking and Alcohol status
- Further to this will be taken a weight history

When you have your first consultation expect, that you are asked many things AND that you ask many things.

I would expect you to have a physical examination that will be undertaken while you are in your underwear.

Many fat people find this an unbearable thought. For many, more often women, it is important to ask for a chaperone to be present. This is usually a nurse. If this is not offered and you feel it is important for you then ASK for one.

You may feel embarrassed, but remember that many have come before you.

Take a deep breath and it will be OK.

I have yet to meet a doctor who notices that you washed your 'good' white bra in with the dark washing! They truly are more interested in listening to your lungs or heart sounds and have come across many a mismatched set of undies. If you are embarrassed by your adipose s/he won't be and as s/he works in the field will be very used to seeing all sorts of shapes and sizes. Try to take it in your stride.

A Nutritionist (Dietician) will ask about your eating habits and foods. Be honest. None of us got fat by eating a lettuce leaf alone ☺ unless we truly have defied science or have some alien within us.

If you were seeing me I would be asking you some questions that would include , for example,

Why do you want surgery and who do you want it for?

I would be asking myself even more questions that may include questions such as is this person ready, willing and able to have a life changing procedure that is no magic wand? Do they truly understand that weight loss surgery is only a tool to help their change? Is this person expecting someone, or something, to do all the work for them? Have they been pushed into asking for surgery, or 'sent' by their GP or medical specialist form another area, but in reality they are happy the shape and size that they are? Is this person going to be open to change?

Such appointments are lengthy and should be of value to you, not only to the health practitioners. Ask yourself some penetrating questions:

- Do I feel safe with them?

- Do I feel comfortable with them?

- Could I work with these people for the long term?

- Do they value and respect me as a person?

- Can I be real and ask them questions?

- Are they being honest with me?

- Are they easy to contact?

It needs courage to ask for help and it needs courage to change.

Well done you are really working hard towards your change.

Private v NHS. Pros and cons

If you are a UK citizen, it is likely that you prefer to use the NHS for your medical care. Once in the NHS patients are reliant on the expertise of those practitioners who are recognised to be some of the best in the world.

The NHS is funded centrally with further, and more local distribution of limited funds. GP consortia, Specialist commissioners are names you may hear.

In some areas the funds are insufficient to support weight loss surgery.

Sadly, as I type this, I have just answered an email from someone who has been recommended by his GP as an ideal candidate for weight loss surgery but the local 'purse holders' say there is no money available.

In some areas funding for weight loss surgery is somewhat limited. Perhaps those who will be 'able to offer society' some financial return e.g. be able to return to work, or continue to work will be a preferred group for surgery. Perhaps those with a very high BMI (50 or over) will be the only patients considered for surgery. None of us know what the future holds for those of us who seek weight loss surgery.

The NHS hospital staff, doctors, managers and nurses have little, if any, influence on this situation. They are often generally sympathetic to the plea of those who have health related conditions that are known to improve with such surgery and will try to support in whatever way they can.

Sadly, in the main their hands remain tied as funding is not made readily available to hospitals and teams who may be able to offer a weight loss surgery service.

Equally, while your GP feels you are highly suitable and motivated he too has little ability to change what is available, or allocated to the National Health Service purse.

Private health care

If you chose to select a private health care provider it is important not to assess on price alone.

There is only 'one of you' and you are worth more than anyone attempting to do a 'hard sell' or glossy magazine drop so, establish facts that will enable you to make an informed choice.

Pile 'em high, sell it cheap, in my opinion is not how one should approach an operation. Please please do not compromise yourself financially, no matter how desperate you are to 'get slim'. The weightloss surgery pathway is life long and costs are equally on going. It is highly, highly, unlikely that you will pay the 'flat fee' as advertised and never need to pay anything more.

As a health practitioner working in the field of weight loss surgery I firmly believe it is essential for anyone contemplating surgery to have a high quality service that includes a full preoperative assessment, extensive investigations and support both during and in the long term following surgery.

Complications occur rarely but if they do happen it is likely to occur between 12 – 18months post operatively and support at this stage is vital.

Obviously, the importance of follow up care, nutritional supplementation and, if necessary, band adjustments are vital to ongoing success and maintenance. If you enter the private sector you will need to consider the finances of the long term not just a 'quick fix' operation. It is essential that you have lifelong follow up available and preferably with the same team who know you and your circumstances.

It is important to remember that in the UK, once a patient within the private sector you are expected to remain in the private sector, unless in the case of an emergency when you are able to attend an NHS hospital.

Think long term - not just an operation day.

Your team

How healthy is the team you are going to be working with?

Do you like them and do you feel safe talking to them?

Do they communicate and have a healthy team attitude between them?

Do they attend study days or team meetings regularly? If you sense in built disharmony or animosity this could impact on your care.

Do you feel this is the right place for you?

In both my professional and personal experience, I have found that relationships between all parties form part of a successful weight loss journey. This begins well before the surgery and, as mentioned previously weight loss surgery is not simply about 'an operation' or a 'quick fix'.

A small percentage of weight GAIN is expected and within approx. 5 years.

Weight loss outcomes are similar between any procedure, be that Gastric bypass or gastric band. No surgery is a 100% guarantee of permanent weight loss and there are many other elements that present over the years, not least the personal changes involved.

I believe it is very important that everyone fully understands the proposed procedure and the long term known effects that any operation will have on eating habits. Also to be aware that there are likely to be unknown long term effects on our bodies.

If not suitable where does the patient go from there?

What if .... you aren't 'fat enough' ?!?

Desperate people can do desperate things and sadly it isn't unknown for some people try to, 'eat their way up' to being fat enough for surgery. Even more sadly they then find even though they are then 'fat enough' no surgery is available in their area on the NHS.

In a place of confusion, anger and disappointment they have begun the Yo Yo scenario again and have now even more of a hurdle to clamber over.

The introduction of a tiered weight loss service in the NHS is likely to be in place where you live. These tiers offer education, nutritional and behavioural therapy and sometimes group work. They have been developed to address the growing 'obesity problem' from as early a stage as possible. It will be interesting to see the outcomes of such services at a 5 or 10 year review.

Sometimes people are offered prescribed medication and 'accountability' type support. At the end of the day the reality is 'It's your choice' what you chose to do and, sadly, getting fatter may be included in that decision.

Those three words – it's your choice! They are so weighted and at times depressing but ... to understand why we chose to 'pop something in our mouth', or eat something in the car and then dispose of the wrappers before we are found out, or hide food where family can't see it .. these are the behaviours we need some support with.

It IS hard work.

Please let me share with you that even when you have weight loss surgery it is hard work to maintain. It is EVEN HARDER to maintain than to lose.

Ways of losing weight non-surgically

Prescribed medication may be helpful for some people but really these are best when combined with other changes including introducing increased activity, food intake and eating behaviour changes.

Some people, who are preparing for weightloss surgery, are encouraged to try (again) something like Xenical to help them lose weight before proceeding to surgery. Some Drs will discuss this with patients at initial assessment.

Prescribed medication should only be considered if 3 months of managed care, involving supervised food intake, managed activity and behavioural change fails to achieve a realistic reduction in weight. Or, for those who have other medical problems such as diabetes, coronary heart disease, high cholesterol, high blood pressure or obstructive sleep apnoea that may increase the risk of e.g. heart disease.

Obviously none of us take medication without really thinking about it and having check ups with the Dr who prescribed it for us in the first place.

What Drugs are Available?

The main drugs available in the UK (at time of writing) for treating obesity is Xenical (Orlistat) ®

Xenical®

Orlistat (Xenical) ® is a drug that reduces the absorption of dietary fat and helps some obese patients lose weight. A 'Lipase inhibitor'. It is now available over the counter as a product called 'Alli' ®

The National Institute for Clinical Excellence have recommended that treatment with Orlistat should only be continued beyond 6 months if at least 10% weight has been lost since the beginning of treatment.

Some of the (positive and negative) effects of Orlistat are:

- Cholesterol levels often improve
- In diabetics, Orlistat can help blood sugar control
- Blood pressure sometimes falls

- Stomach cramps, wind, oily leakage from the rectum, liquid or oily stools, faecal incontinence and diarrhoea - however these symptoms are usually mild and get better after the first few weeks of treatment.

What are the surgical options? Pros and cons

Simon will discuss the surgery in greater depth in a later chapter. However, as a female, and as a 'bandee' I like to get my "two pennith" in!

Surgery is a serious option. It is not a 'cosmetic' procedure, although sometimes it is advertised as being so.

An advert in the female part of a newspaper, or at the back of a glossy magazine, does not truly equate the significance of having surgery.

Weight loss surgery is an operation, as much as having your gall bladder removed. Having a general anaesthetic holds a risk factor for those who are not obese and the risks are increased if someone is obese.

When we are fat we focus, in the main, on 'being thin'. I'll do whatever ... I don't care ... it means I will be thin ....are things I often have said to me.

I guess it's the same as many things in our lives; parenthood, marriage, profession... we believe, in the main it will be good, perhaps have difficult times but not very difficult.

I want it to happen ... 'now', yesterday, tomorrow, in a few months. So the desire to 'be thin' can, and does, for some of us somehow 'over ride' the 'common sense' part of our brains.

Would you buy a car, buy a house, move house, have an extension built or start a new career without asking people, researching comparing and then mulling the pros and cons over? I very much doubt it and yet, our overriding desire to 'have' or to 'be' thin blinkers us to a fixed route at times.

Personal opinion - The surgeons I work with are great.

It would be a sad story if after all these years I thought otherwise! Equally I recognise that they are mere mortals. They get upset, moody, have migraines, prang their cars, go on holiday where it rains all the time, get fat, get thin, probably ignore someone's birthday (I'll pass my date to them now!) They don't claim to be 'the best in the world, or two of the best in the country' (although on a personal level I feel they fit the latter category!!) but they are equally not full of the 'surgeon hormone'!

'Surgeon hormone' is a very old hormone discovered many years ago and can present along the lines of:-

- 'I'm a surgeon, I know best, I am the best and I will 'cure you'.

- 'You may have questions and I will tell you

what the answers are and what you have to do'.

- 'You are fat if you have this operation (and I've done thousands) you will only need to take a vitamin tablet a day and, 'Bob's your Uncle' your thin dream will be with you and ...... I will be your hero'.

Have you met the type?

Your head comes out of the consultation spinning. Your body follows exhaustedly behind. Your 'being slender' dreams are closer and being slender equals .... whatever it means for you.

Thankfully, we work as a team and there are no supermen expounding the greatness of how surgery can be a 'cure all'. The truth is, it isn't.

NONE of us live with your surgery 24/7 ONLY you do this and as such you need to know what is likely to be the result of surgery on a day to day basis.

All surgery has other factors to consider and include possible impact on the lungs, heart and blood vessels and in some cases psychological complications. In addition to familiar things such as 'infection' it is perhaps useful to know that with weight loss surgery 10 to 20 percent of patients who have weight-loss surgery require follow-up operations to correct complications of varying types.

Chapter 6

PREPARING FOR THE OP

What on earth am I doing?

Is it really worth all the soul searching and waiting? The feeling of dread, someone putting a foreign object in place where there should be none. The realisation, this sleep may be my final one.

I guess, on the positive side, death means no ironing, no picking up 'stuff' from the floor and no cleaning the reoccurring rim around the bath every day.

The flip side, not feeling warm sun on my face, kicking leaves in the Autumn or tasting fresh new potatoes from the garden. Worst of all, never to feel the touch of my children again, never to hear their voices, or listen to them play the piano or even argue!

I would be the grandma who isn't there and died young,

"of course she was very fat, very fat, so none of us were surprised".

I know I am more likely to die the shape and size I am than during the operation. Even so what on earth am I doing? Is it really, really worth it?

All this because ….because I've tried everything and I'm too fat, I've eaten too much for whatever reason.

It's simple…………..I am doing it for me. I am worth it and I am worth more than remaining the same.

I want to be able to reach my feet, clip my nails and paint them a 'tarty' red! I want to book flights and not have to worry about the size of the seatbelt or the 'orange extension'. I want to go to a restaurant or café and not be filled with dread when every chair has arms or if the seats are 'fixed' to the floor with little, if any, room to fit. I want to be able to eat a meal without the world and his wife staring at me.

I want to go shopping in high street clothes store just like everybody else does and walk up and down the aisles with an arm full of clothes to try on. I want them to have the 'wow' factor and not always be various shades of the black and navy. I want to walk into the changing rooms without the willow thin assistant looking at me with the look that says, 'who are you kidding thinking that'll fit you!?'

I want to try clothes on without going to the 'fat lady shop' where I try all the clothes on only to see my bra through the gaping large arm holes – why do designers think all fat people have fat arms? I don't know.

I don't want to experience, 'it fits so I had better buy it' shopping trip any more.

I want to get into a car and slip into the space in front of the steering wheel, not be worried that the seat belt cuts into my neck because my 'top half' is so large the belt simply has nowhere to go but 'upwards'!

I want to climb a flight of stairs and not gasp like a chronic asthmatic half way up. I want to be able to walk up a hill without stopping to catch my breath every few minutes. I want to go for a walk and not think about the aches of tomorrow.

I want to kneel in the garden and be able to get up again without my back hurting.

I want to enjoy life instead of conducting a risk assessment for potential embarrassing moments of everything I do.

I want a future when I can plan wonderful holidays and family events and not think of my family planning my funeral. I want to pick up my grandchildren from school without their friends saying, 'your grandma is fat'.

None of my family want me to have this operation. They love me as I am and are fearful that I may die. Yet I am likely to die because of my size. I sure don't like the shape and size that I am I don'.

That summarises some of the reasons why I want a band. I want the 'outside fatter me' to shrink and meet the 'inside thinner me'.

When they become one I am excited to know how it will feel and what changes I will feel. It's peculiar to think of a smaller sized me - less visible less observed.

READY?

Change can be messy, scary and uncomfortable for any of us. I think that's why so many of us chose to remain the same, not to introduce change into our lives. We can feel safe even in the most uncomfortable situations. Familiarity may breed contempt but equally it may equal soft fuzzy safety that does not demand change, or so we may think.

Such a radical change of body shape and size can be both exciting and daunting.

Imagine, only a few years ago I knew someone who I thought was a 'perfect' shape and size - whatever that it?! She had 'stuff' in her life, as is often the case. A bumpy relationship, two children and she ran her own busy but successful business.

Sadly she was truly 'hung up' about her 'saddle bags'.

Frankly, I had difficulty in identifying where the alleged offending adipose lay. However, for her it was devastating. Her saddle bags were a huge, if not THE huge problem in her life. She decided to have liposuction. The change mechanism kicked in.

As a size 'expletive' I guess you'd love merely to have saddle bags and not the rest! Even so, if you were the svelte woman with saddle bags (sorry chaps) considering surgery it's change. Contemplation, realisation, dreams, hopes, future visualisation, anxiety, concern, fear, questioning etc etc.

No one knows how it will work out. Will the sites become infected? Will the scars be worse than the saddle bags? No one can predict the future. No one knows how being banded will work out or if the impact will be as imagined.

Incidentally, she had the liposuction, was thrilled to bits however, her world didn't improve. Her relationship collapsed, as did her business. 'Stuff' continued to happen to her even without saddlebags.

So ask yourself the two 'R's - 'am I Really Ready'.

You won't be able to sit back for this journey, you won't be the spectator on the sidelines you will be 'dug in' for the long haul and there will be days you will want to escape from the reality and the possible battles you will experience with 'you'. 'Stuff' will still happen whatever shape and size you are and it's not always positive 'stuff'!

Being 'surrounded in adipose' can oddly be very reassuring and safe for some of us. Outsiders can't quite 'reach' us or 'touch' us physically in quite the same way. The same applies at an emotional level for some of us.

I have some patients who freely tell me that emotionally being fat is a very comfortable, protective and familiar place. They don't like the outer body and battle so hard, like a tortoise trying to shed its shell.

Sometimes, to put it simply, chose to remain as they are.

For whatever reason, being as we are can serve us. No matter how much hard work it is to lug an 'additional weight' around, clothe it and bathe it for some it may have some positives attached.

I hear you say, 'you must be off your tree'!

Think about it. One dear lady told me how she loved the fact that her size meant that she could not easily get out of bed. Her 13 year old daughter spent quality time with her mother by bringing her food.

Another gentle single chap in his 30's could not leave his flat and could barely walk. His loneliness was relieved by his sister doing his shopping and cooking meals for him.

The 'love language' of food and feeding is so important for many of us and so abused at times.

Please, please, remember, it is truly not a crime to choose to stay as you are - if this is where you want to be.

So, are the changes 'Really Really' worth it to you?

WILLING?

OK, this is going to be a little 'blunt' and you may want to throw this book across the room in a moment!

If you feel that you are the shape and size you are for an unknown reason then please do not have surgery.

Sadly, unless you are an alien, have broken the known laws of Physics, or have some extremely rare genetic condition, the reason you are the size you are is because too much fuel is going into your body for your energy needs.

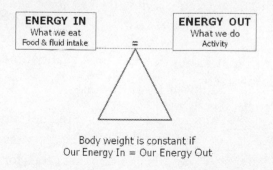

My loathed energy equation

Loathed because, as many others, I would like to eat exactly what I want to in the volumes I want to eat it in. I have had to grow up and accept the fact too much on my lips equals more inches on my hips. The rebellious child part of me is now stamping my foot and saying, 'it's not fair!'

After over 10 years of being banded I still struggle with this however I was willing to change and am still willing to learn more about myself and my reactions. I may not always like what I learn but I have had to be willing to mature emotionally and reason with myself a little more.

How many of us want to take ourselves outside and 'work ourselves over' having eaten 'that'? Instead of beating yourself up and condemning yourself when you have eaten 'that' how about asking yourself, 'am I willing to be nice to me'?

So many of us, are only too keen to continually think disparagingly about ourselves. Does this result in anything positive? I can't remember who said it, probably someone very famous, '*if your treat your friends as you treat yourself you would have very few friends*'.

How about lightening up on you?

Are you willing to accept that you need to think about you?

I have met patients who feel they are so unique they are

beyond help. Nothing can, has, or will ever 'work' for them. Somehow this group of people have little willingness to introduce change. They are not willing to work 100% and expect something, or someone, to do all the work.

Guess what, sometimes their self fulfilling prophecy becomes reality. There are a small population of patients who genuinely want to prove to everyone they are so very unique and different they chose to sabotage themselves, and the band, by 'pushing' their food and fluid intake.

I'd never do that. How silly when you have had an operation to help me. Believe me we all try it at times. However most of us are willing to knuckle down and look at what we are doing.

Of course if you truly fall into this category you're setting yourself up for failure and a fair few wasted years of fighting with yourself and your band.

Don't bother, honestly, just buy the postcard and imagine that you had been there.

Are you willing to introduce significant behavioural change into your life for the rest of your life?

When the initial honeymoon period subsides and the realisation that it is hard work and costly to stay a smaller size are you willing to continue to pick your feet up to walk through this part of your life.

Are you willing to accept that some people who you believe are your nearest and dearest may actually like you as you are and chose therefore to (probably subconsciously) attempt to sabotage your efforts to hold you where your are.

Listen up reader, there are partners out there who will want to pop out to 'the garage' for some nibbles at 9pm. There are chronic feeders living with some of us. There are the Passive Aggressive partners who we allow to push us to the end and then we heal with food, or drink. None of us 'have to buy' crisps, biscuits or chocolate to keep in the house for our children. Good excuse but cut it out!

You may be living with one of the above or with one of the classic excuses of why you 'have' to buy junk.

Moving to the surgery, are you willing to accept that you may have complications?

Are you willing to accept that you may need to have more surgery or, that you may not be happy with the physical change and psychological work?

All surgery brings with it a chance of the need to have more surgery, as Simon will explain.

www.avonobesityservice.co.uk

http://obesitysurgery-info.com/wls_release_form.htm

ABLE??

I know you are able to do the most amazing things in your life.

Perhaps this is the only area where you have hit 'the wall', the pain barrier. Even if you have, in the past, and will possibly hit it again in the future, that no way means that you are not able.

Are you able to recognise why you use food and eating when not linked to hunger?

Are you able to recognise and understand food and eating related coping strategies? If you are able to recognise these familiar behaviours it is likely that you are able to change them. Perhaps with professional help and perhaps not.

I feel sure that most of you reading this do have the personal resources to begin and sustain this new weight loss journey.

As with many things is life planning, preparation and realistic goals are key. If you were going for a walk on Dartmoor you would, I hope, be prepared for many possible eventualities – this is no different.

If you can honestly say yes to most of the points then think now about life with a band, eating living and socialising.

Decide to decide

When you have decided to 'go for it' there is likely to be a period of waiting. Use this as preparation time. You could sit and wait for 'it' to happen however, you're going to have to make some changes in eating soon so why not action some things in preparation during those long days you are counting.

If you always do what you've always done then you'll always get what you've always got.

So, when you are ready decide to decide to change.

Kathy, our nutritionist, suggests some of these points as a pre-op time filler.

Slow down your eating rate.

Do you 'bolt' your food?

It actually takes about 20 minutes for your brain to register that you have had sufficient fuel. If you eat quickly you can get through a lot of food in that time!

Next time you are out having a coffee watch other people eat and drink.

Do they put their knives and forks down between mouthfuls? Do they chew their food? Do they finish after a few minutes?

Now try timing you and your family meal times.

Since being banded I have a real problem with rushed meal times. Not only because with a band you simply cannot rush but also because I value the ambience, the company, eating and quality of food much more than prior to banding.

Small portions of high quality well prepared food is my ideal now.

It makes me so sad that I have spent hours thinking about, buying and preparing a wonderful meal only for it to be consumed in a few minutes. If I asked my husband what we had eaten for lunch he wouldn't have had a clue, 'sausages' would be his random guess.

All my hard work ….. for hurried and un-chewed mouthfuls and the table cleared within less time than it took me to prepare. Why did I get up early to prepare for a lovely Sunday Roast? Why did I go over budget to buy the special joint of meat for Sunday? Why did I make such a superb pudding for it all to be gone in a few seconds?

How long does it take you to prepare a meal? Now ask how long does it take to eat what you have prepared. Are you valuing you, the food and your effort? Less than 10 minutes eating I suggest is a bit of an insult to your thoughtful preparation and hard work. Less than 10 minutes and your body has barely had time to log that you are eating.

Other people have found some of these tips helpful:

- Chewing each mouthful at least 20 times *(Even people who've had a band for a long time say that they still get caught out by eating too fast and not chewing their food well enough)*

- Eat only when you are sitting down at a table – no TV and no reading to distract you. Try using baby cutlery of chopsticks to help you slow down.

Eat mindfully.

My mother has told me of her years as a war time young person living in London. Rationing, having an orange for the first time. How precious and the taste was unique.

Imagine, when you eat, that this is the only food available for the foreseeable future. Value it, taste it, smell it you may never see or have this food again.

Focus only on what you are eating – remember it is precious.

- How does it taste? What texture is it? Is it more enjoyable to bite and chew it than simply letting it slip away? Does it depend on your mood?

One thing at a time.

How many people do we see each day walking with a cardboard cup in hand, eating as they walk to work. While we are able to multi task in many things we really need not 'eat on our feet'.

Would we be so mindless in our eating if food were less readily available, if this were likely to be our only food available for the foreseeable future? Would we devalue food and eating if it were rationed once again? Would we drive and eat if that one sandwich was all that there was available for the foreseeable future?

Try to concentrate on the wonders of the fuel we have. Honour your body by allowing it to taste and digest and enjoy the pleasure of eating with thought.

Portion sizes

You only need to type in 'portion distortion' into the www and you will see how portion sizes have increased over recent years. We take it as 'normal' to see a large plate overfilled. I would certainly have sought that in the past. Believe me I am no saint now and my 'size eyes' sometimes make a bid to be heard. When you are banded you simply won't be able to cope with large portions of hurried food so think about it now.

Someone once suggested serving your usual meal onto two plates. Eat the first plate slowly then wait 20 minutes.

When you have waited ask yourself, 'do I really need that second plate full?'

You can think about using a smaller plate, or buy a plate with a wide border pattern making sure your meal stays within the border.

Whatever ticks the box for you and works for you run with it for the length of season it works for.

Permission to leave.

I give you full permission to leave food on your plate.

Indeed you may become a 'no longer a member of the clean plate club'.

No one will chastise you, you are now an adult. You won't be presented with it at breakfast or at any other time, unless you do that to yourself. No one will starve if you leave food on your plate. Anyway, who, in this country would want to eat your half eaten cold food anyway?

Of course logically, if you cooked less you'd serve less ☺

Food groups

Here I should, I guess, sound wise and intelligent! I should ask if you are eating adequate protein, vitamins and carbohydrates. In reality there are a number of malnourished and significantly overweight people.

Many experience food cravings if they are low micro nutrients or minerals. So, check out what food types you eat.

Start to be aware of what your food is like just before you swallow it.

When you have a band, you need to make sure that you have chewed food to the right texture. Almost like baby food, before swallowing it. If you do not do this it may cause pain and a blockage.

Start to be aware of what your food is like just before you swallow it. If it's not porridge texture or baby food texture, you need to chew it some more!

Here are some foods to experiment with:

- Try a banana. At the moment, you probably want to swallow it when it is a mixture of 'smoothie' texture and some lumps. Chew it a bit more until it is completely smooth. Bananas are actually often difficult foods for a banded person to eat.

- Try some granary or wholemeal bread. You probably want to swallow it when it is in a doughy ball. Chew it some more until it is at the soggy sloppy stage.

- Cut a tomato into pieces. Can you manage to chew it to a pureed stage?

- Try a mouthful of roast or casseroled meat. What stage was it at when you wanted to swallow? How much more did you have to chew to get it to a pureed stage?

Are you actually hungry or is it a craving?

Many people who come to see us say they aren't sure if they know what hunger feels like. You might be interpreting a 'head hunger' or emotional emptiness as physical hunger. Here are some things you can try to check if you're really hungry:

True hunger comes on like waves on a beach. It moves in and out. Emotional hunger is more often like a thunder clap from nowhere!

- Some people confuse thirst with hunger. Try a glass of water first.

- If that doesn't help, do you want more of something you've already eaten? If the answer is 'no' then you're not hungry. You may simply want to echo the taste.

- Did you only start wanting the food because you'd seen it or smelled it – or even thought about it? In which case, it's a craving.

- Cravings start to lessen in 20 minutes. What could you do to distract yourself for 20 minutes?

- Other people have done things like brushing their teeth, painting their nails, cleaning the kitchen cupboards and surfaces or doing something on the computer.

Start to think about why you over-eat

If you have a band it does nothing other than slow your eating down and reduce your portion size. Would that it were a brain transplant at times but ... it isn't and all the familiar feelings, thoughts and emotions that trigger your overeating will still be there. Which is why it is good to practice before you have an operation. The operation won't do this bit for you.

Are you eating because you're bored / fed-up / upset / stressed?

What else could you do when you feel this way?

Kick something (not somebody), open the washing machine and shout into it – yes I have done that one! Personally I couldn't put together a 'kit' or box of things I like doing but some people do.

You probably find a 'full-up' feeling is comforting.

How long does this comfort last? What else gives you this comforted feeling?

Are you eating because the food is there?

You may be highly geared and sensitive to food and eating cues. Seeing, smelling or even simply knowing that your trigger foods are 'behind that door'.

Some tell me that the most effective way round this is to do some planning and change your surroundings and routines to reduce your exposure to cues to eat. Personally I have to use the avoidance trick – i.e. don't buy huge amounts of cheese!

What is stopping you keeping only 'friendly' foods in the house? Do you really need to bulk buy?

Could you go shopping or stop for petrol when you've just eaten rather than when you are hungry?

Can you alter your routine so that you avoid tempting situations?

Could you find another route rather than passing the bakery?

Are these real reasons or excuses?

Look at the sequence of events that leads to you over-eating.

This is SUCH hard work but very interesting to unpick!

What were you thinking or feeling beforehand.

Did that affect your decision to eat?

Is there another way of looking at these things?

Many people use food and eating as their coping mechanism. How will you cope if food is taken away?

You may, at some stage decide that you need some professional help with this one. If you do then 'run; with it. It's hard work, can be expensive if not funded by the NHS but it may well help you unpick your relationship with food and eating.

Start to think about your previous attempts to lose weight and what you can learn from them.

You're probably very good at losing weight and can easily recall when you lost 3 stone on the xx diet and show the photo of when you were a fleeting size 'teeny tiny'. However you may not yet found the answer to *maintaining* your food and eating changes.

It may be helpful to think through what happened that stopped you doing something that was originally successful. Often it isn't just one thing but several things happening at around the same time.

For example, many people say they were following a set

diet and then lapsed. The voice in your head then started to tell you you'd blown it and were never going to be successful so you might as well…….

And then you started to think that you were fed up anyway of eating salads. And also, you hated having to be organised and plan what you ate. And it was Christmas and it wasn't fair that you couldn't eat the 'nice foods'.

And before very long you'd talked yourself out of continuing!

Many people describe themselves as 'all or nothing' people and either do something to extremes or not at all.

Is it possible you're setting yourself up for failure by setting very rigid dietary rules that no-one could keep to? Who says you have to eat salads to lose weight? Why can't you eat nice foods and still lose weight?

Think about what support you can enlist for making these changes

Most people say that having support is a great help. Whose support could you rely on when the going gets tough? Family? A supportive friend? Someone who will listen?

Think about life after you've had the Band.

Many people find after the operation that there are foods

they can't manage. How will you feel if you can never eat certain foods (such as bread) again?

How will your family cope with you being able to eat only very small amounts?

Will it affect your family meals?

If it takes you a long time to eat, how will you manage at work?

What will you do about social occasions: meals out, special occasions, holidays, a visit to the pub?

Are there people who might attempt to 'sabotage' your attempts? What will you do about that?

Set yourself <u>small</u> goals for changes

Goals need to be SMART:

Specific,

Measurable,

Achievable,

Realistic / Relevant

Time-limited

For example: I will never eat puddings again isn't a SMART goal (not realistic!).

I will eat fruit instead of pudding once next week *is* a SMART goal

I will do more exercise isn't SMART (not specific or measurable).

I will go to the gym every day isn't SMART (probably not achievable!)

I will walk to work once next week is SMART

Remember Rome wasn't built in a day!

Chapter 7

IMMEDIATELY PRE-OP

You may be asked to attend the endoscopy department pre-operatively.

Endoscopy

Endoscopy is one of the necessary evils that has to be endured to be able to proceed to the next stage of the banding journey. Not the most pleasant way of spending an afternoon but necessary all the same.

It involves a trained doctor putting a thin flexible tube down into the oesophagus, stomach and small intestine that has a fibre-optic light at the end of it. Any abnormalities can be clearly seen.

Before going to the clinic the stomach has to be empty so there is no eating or drinking, including water for at least six hours beforehand. On arrival an endoscopy nurse patiently explains all that is going to happen and what the options are as far as sedation goes.

A light sedative anaesthetic can be given and most patients do not remember the procedure when the effects wear off. The disadvantage of this is the inability to leave swiftly and drive home afterwards for dinner! Oh and you aren't insured for the following twenty four hours.

The other alternative is to have the back of the throat sprayed with a local anaesthetic which tastes fishy but prevents excessive gagging as the tube is passed down.

Opting for no sedation but with the proviso that if not tolerating the procedure you can change your mind is often the preferred route. My throat was sprayed and a mouth guard placed in my mouth. I was laid on my left side in a darkened room and once I was comfortable the endoscope was passed through my mouth. Annoyingly, my back was towards the monitor so I was unable to have a conducted tour of my digestive tract.

I would be lying if I said it was the most comfortable procedure, who knows what I would chose if I ever had to have it done again. I guess it would depend on many reasons including if I had to drive the next day. It could not have lasted more than a few minutes.. Eventually the tube reached my small intestine and the doctor told me that he was coming back up again. I took this to mean that the tube would be removed imminently but he continued to carefully examine every nook and cranny in thorough detail.

Once the tube was removed and given the news that I was anatomically normal I was allowed to leave after a short while in the waiting room to ensure I had no adverse reaction.

Pre op assessment. What to expect

The pre-surgery week of yoghurt is hard, very hard and even the most determined patient is reported to have 'a slip' during the week. Choose low fat or fat free varieties in as many flavours as possible and space the pots out through the day.

Plan the day carefully so that there is always something to look forward or somewhere to go even if it is only the local library or shops. This takes the mind away from eating and while you are shopping you can't eat. Don't plan to meet friends in places that food is readily available. Explain to them what the yoghurt week is all about and they will be supportive. Go to the cinema, knit a jumper or do a jigsaw.

DON'T go to the supermarket unless absolutely necessary. The smell of the fresh bread coming out of the oven in the bakery section will only be torture. Send another family member with a shopping list.

Prepare meals for the rest of the family the week beforehand so that you do not have to cook for the week pre and post surgery.

Use the support from family, friends, colleagues etc. They will all be behind you helping you to get through the week.

Look on this week as a challenge. I felt that if I could not get through it then it was indicative that I did not want the band as much as I thought I did. If I could cope with seven days of yoghurt then I could cope with anything that was in front of me. It is also a great way to loose weight before surgery and there is nothing like watching the scales going down each day to give that extra motivation.

By following the 'diet', the liver will reduce in size so making surgery easier. One of the functions of the liver is to storing a form of sugar known as glycogen so that when the body needs glucose these stores can be called upon to release energy. For every ounce of glycogen the body will store 3-4 ounces of water. By restricting your daily input to six pots of low fat yoghurt causes the liver to release water and glycogen to provide energy to other organs resulting in the liver reducing in size. As the body's store of water is also being reduced it is necessary to maintain fluid levels during this week to prevent dehydration.

Right, I think you're now ready for your op!

Chapter 8

THE OPERATION

Congratulations! You've made it through to the day of surgery. All those months of deliberating, appraising and accepting are over. You are probably feeling excited, stressed, nervous, hungry – all of these thoughts and feelings are to be expected and most importantly, are normal. I will explain in this chapter the course of events that will occur over the next 48hrs in order to allay your fears and reassure you that you are in very safe hands.

On the morning of surgery, you will be on a ward. You will be greeted by the team of doctors and nurses who will be looking after you and the first thing to realise is that they are experienced. You are not the first gastric band patient they have looked after and you won't be the last so trust in them and let them do the worrying for you. After all the routine checks (blood pressure, pulse, temperature etc.) have been completed, you will be asked to sign a consent form. This is a very important legal document which highlights the risks and benefits of the surgery. It tells you what complications are possible, although unlikely. This information should not be new to you if the system has worked well as you should have been fully counselled on your journey up to this point. Don't feel under pressure to sign this immediately as it is important that you have digested all the information and are ready to commit to the next phase of your journey. The likelihood though, is that you will be champing at the bit to get it signed.

Next comes the dress code – hospital gowns, net knickers and tight stockings – agreed not the most attractive of outfits but trust me, the stockings can be a life-saver. They encourage blood flow in the legs and help prevent deep vein thrombosis (DVT) – so don't put up resistance when the sister insists you wear them. Do what you are told – remember they are looking after you now.

When it comes to the time for surgery, most places encourage you to walk to theatre. This is to empower you and make you feel less like a "patient" being wheeled on a trolley down long corridors. Its amazing the difference it makes and you should embrace this exercise as over the next few days you will most probably not feel like doing a great deal.

When you come through into the theatre complex you will arrive in the holding bay where you will be registered. Shortly you will go to the anaesthetic room where you will be re-united with the anaesthetic team (lovingly referred to as the "gas-board"). They will explain to you, again, what will happen as you drift off to sleep. Again, to empower you, you will be asked to walk into theatre and position yourself on the operating table. Now, the theatre can be a daunting place but actually most of the time, I find it a really special place to be. There are lots of people all with differing roles but more often than not these people are smiling, chatty and always ready to crack a joke. Theatres run like clockwork, everyone knows what they are doing so don't be scared – feel privileged to be part of this team.

Next you will receive some drugs through the drip in your arm and you will calmly drift off to sleep. Almost certainly the anaesthetist will support your chin and hold an oxygen mask over your face as this is happening to ensure that your breathing is optimum. When you are asleep, they will then place a tube in your throat to help take over your breathing when you are asleep. Don't worry, you will not be aware of this happening.

Next the surgeons take over. There will be a lead surgeon (usually the consultant) and several experienced assistants, all of whom are highly trained. They will take responsibility for your positioning on the table. You will be tilted to an angle of forty five degrees so that access to your stomach is made easier – gravity is the surgeon's friend here. At all times, your dignity will be preserved. You will have discreetly placed towels over your bits and every effort will be made to ensure that you are treated with respect and humanity, as if you were awake.

Your tummy will then be "prepped" – painted with a golden brown antiseptic iodine based solution. Once this has been thoroughly done and rigorously checked, you will then be "draped" – putting sterile towels around the edges of the field of operating. Once this has been done, it's lights, camera, action!

All equipment will have been checked and tested. The surgeon will then inflate your tummy with gas (carbon dioxide) to allow space for the key-hole instruments - the idea being that the abdominal muscle wall is lifted away from the organs by a cushion of gas. This is achieved using a long blunt needle (Verres needle) which is inserted just under the ribs on your left hand side. Once the tummy is inflated to the right pressure, the operating can start. Several "ports" are then inserted into abdominal muscle wall and these will allow various instruments, a camera and the gastric band to be passed in and out multiple times.

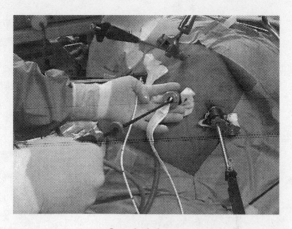

An inflated abdomen with
instrument ports demonstrated.

Once the ports are in place the operation can proceed. The liver is held out of the way to improve access to the stomach. This is where the yoghurt diet comes in and is so vital. This diet shrinks the size of the liver considerably to make surgery easier. In fact sometimes, surgery can't proceed if the liver is too big. Remember, big on the outside, means big on the inside too. The liver accumulates and stores fat and will get bigger as weight increases so any pre-operative attempt to lose weight will be appreciated by your surgeon, trust me!

Next, once the liver is safely out of the way, a space is created around the top of the stomach just below where the food pipe joins the stomach. This is where the band will sit. Once this space has been created, it's time to put in the band. This is a highly engineered, sophisticated bit of kit and the surgeon will take very good care of it during the procedure. Sterility will be of the utmost importance to keep germs out. The following picture shows a gastric band. The tube attached and the metal port are to allow inflation and deflation of the internal reservoir of the band to tighten or loosen it. This will become a very familiar process to you over the next few weeks, to months.

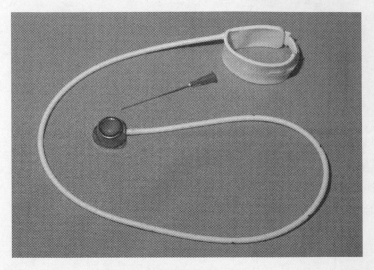

A gastric band (MIDband™) with inflation / deflation port attached.

The band will be placed around the upper stomach and fastened in position. The band is often stitched in position by the surgeon but this is certainly not necessary and will be down to individual surgeon choice.

The tubing is brought out onto the surface of your abdominal wall and the metal port is attached. This is then buried in the fat of your abdominal wall or stitched to your muscle wall; again different techniques are practiced in different places but excellent results can be expected either way. This port needs to be accessible to your team, long into the future so that the band can be adjusted without further surgery.

The operation then finishes with a quick re-check inside to make sure that all is well and then the wounds from the ports are closed with dissolvable stitches. You will have up to six small key holes wounds in your upper abdomen which will fade quickly over the coming months.

After the operation, you will be tidied up and then taken to recovery, where you will be gently and calmly woken up from your deep sleep. You will feel drowsy and maybe a little disorientated but the nurses here, will constantly reassure you until you are "back in the room".

When the recovery team are happy with your progress you will be taken back to the ward where you will begin your journey as a "banded" person. This really is the moment that you take control and start your new life. It will take hard work and you will have your down days but it will be so worth it, I promise.

You may have an x-ray on the first day afterwards to check the positioning of the band and once you are able to take liquids by mouth you will be counseled about your new life with the band so there should be no unanswered questions. Patients are full of questions usually about how to eat and what to eat but this will be fully explained by the dietician and the rest of the team. You should leave with a sense of achievement, a sense of well-being and enormous anticipation about the next steps.

What can go wrong?

The answer is truthfully anything but reassuringly the majority of times, is nothing. Bleeding is often a nuisance for the surgeon rather than a major problem but in cases of brisk bleeding, the surgeon is trained to calmly deal with this. If bleeding cannot be quickly stopped with key hole techniques, then the surgeon may decide to open your abdomen with a large incision to gain quick control of the situation. This is vanishing rare.

The other rare problem is damage to the bowel. The surgeon is operating around your stomach and close to the intestines and it is theoretically possible to make a small hole in any of these structures. Most of the time these are easily sorted by a simple stitch but, as in the case of heavy bleeding, a big incision on your tummy may become necessary. Sometimes small holes in the bowel are not immediately obvious and become apparent over the next few days - this will require a trip back to theatre to put things right. It is important that you know about these things BUT as I said, they are rare. The majority of times, there will be no problem and you will sail through your operation.

The other concern for you and your surgeon is blood clots

in the legs. You don't need to do the worrying, you just need to do what you're told! We take great care over this aspect of your care. Before your operation you will receive a blood thinning injection which will help prevent clots. During the operation, you will be wearing those "o-so-attractive" stockings and you will have special calve pumps which will intermittently pump blood back up your legs to your heart. Post –operatively, you will have your blood thinning injections (for two weeks – you will be trained to do these at home) and you will be encouraged to get out of bed and walk. No languishing in bed – it's time to be pro-active!

In the longer term, you can experience problems but with the right package of after-care these should be minimal. I'll just take a few moments to mention in passing some of the problems that can occur but do bare in mind, these are rare. The biggest problem, that we as surgeons, worry about is something called, "slippage". (See following pictures) When a band "slips", the stomach below the band pushes up through the band and causes the small pouch above to become rapidly bigger. This can, in the worst case scenario, put pressure on the stomach wall, cutting off its blood supply and resulting in a perforation. This can be very serious and will require urgent surgery. Most slips are less serious, thankfully, and can be managed by immediate band deflation and rest for several weeks. Sometimes, the band needs to be unfastened by another operation so that the stomach can return to its normal position and then this can be sorted out several weeks down the line with band repositioning and refastening. The main cause for a slip is excessive vomiting or failure to follow the strict dietary regimes post-operatively. Symptoms include drooling of saliva, an inability to swallow and keep down liquids. These symptoms should alert you to the fact there is trouble and you should seek immediate help either through GP or by presenting to Accident & Emergency.

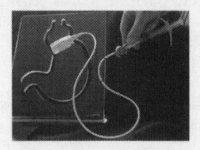

Correct band positioning

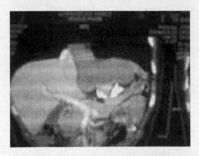

A "Slippage" (note the band is now horizontal as opposed to angled and the small pouch above the band has enlarged)

Other problems include "band failure" where there is no weight loss and no restriction. This can be for a number of reasons, most often due to technical aspects of the band system. There can be a leak in the internal reservoir balloon or in the tubing so that the balloon is deflated. If this is the case, I'm afraid it's another operation to replace it. Sometimes the balloon can be damaged during the operation either by stitching needles or damage as it travels through the ports. This type of damage is not always immediately obvious.

Another worry, but thankfully rare, is an "erosion" - this is where the gastric band slowly over many months starts to burrow its way through the stomach wall so that part of it ends up on the inside. The most common way this presents is putting on weight as the band becomes ineffective. We have means of dealing with it and sometimes this can be sorted out by endoscopy (a camera down the gullet) rather than a separate operation. If this is the case, then re-banding is not always appropriate and you may be offered a different type of weight loss procedure once recovered.

One final thing to remember, as you lose weight, your skin will almost certainly become saggy forming an apron around your middle. You may be inclined to seek plastic surgery to remove this excess skin, but currently this is not funded in the NHS, except in exceptional circumstances. This may be the first operation of a series for you.

Anyway, that's enough of that. Complications are rare. Focus on the positives. Go on, enjoy your new life. Sharon will now explain what happens after the band and how you reach your Shangri-La.

Chapter 9

POST SURGERY – EMOTIONAL ROLLER COASTER

The experience of surgery

My experience of surgery was good, in fact much easier than I had imagined.

Immediate post surgery – physical

Post surgery – physical

'Done and dusted' – I'm a 'new person', now I'm going to be thin! (Hmmmmmmm)

The following morning I was taken for an X-ray (you

sip and swallow fluid). Not everywhere does this but the centre I went to does.

I chatted with the dietician and discussed food intake for the next few days and then, at last, a cup of tea. One that had never tasted so good!

I was ready to go home, apart from being taught to inject myself daily for ten days – a treatment to prevent the formation of blood clots. I hadn't expected this, am not a 'medical' person but just about coped with it.

My previous experience of surgery has been an emergency Caesarean section. Although many years younger, at that time, I found that experience to be painful and I took a long time to recover. I guess having a new baby to care for at the same time didn't help.

Being banded is absolutely nothing in comparison. I have been told that being banded is also less painful than a gall bladder removal or hernia repair.

I experienced some discomfort rather than 'pain'. A dissolvable Paracetamol dealt with any slight discomfort and I think I only took about 2 doses anyway.

New rules of the road

Clearly I had been supported in understanding changes that were to come. Thankfully these tend to be slow changes and easier to cope with. In my head I realised that there would be times of frustration and that it wasn't going to be a magical solution to my long term issues and disease. I had spent hours reading, researching and taking to people. I thought I knew how I would need to chew food and to learn to recognise a 'different' understanding of 'no longer in need of fuel' – 'full'

In theory, you will be 'ready', well prepared and willing. However, as everyone knows, theory is often different from practice.

How can you truly know how it will feel, or how you will feel and react when, 'they' are eating chips and you can't get even one chip down'.

Post op reflection

The Honeymoon

Initially, post-op the 'honeymoon high' can be almost exhilarating. Lack of desire to eat, an underlying 'be safe / be cautious' can be wonderful. However, after a couple of weeks – you may want to 'test' your band and may be shocked, even panic stricken, that you can pretty much each what you could before.

Ok so you eat more slowly and in smaller quantities but many wonder if they have 'done' something. It's unusual if there is anything 'wrong'. Put simply, 'that's just how it is'. Having said that, we are all different and some people do not experience the ability to eat in this way. That's OK too!

Just go with the flow, relax, it is doubtful that you are 'doing anything wrong'.

The self-admonishment, metaphorically beating yourself up with wet spaghetti will achieve little apart from repeating your old behaviours and coping strategies.

Common themes at this point include:

- *I can eat anything* - What am I doing wrong?

- *Something's not right because I believed I wouldn't be 'able' to eat* - Has my band slipped?

- *I don't feel 'full'* – My band isn't 'working'? – Reality ALERT – have you ever felt 'full' or recognised true hunger.

- *Why am I different?* – Special person ALERT – you are no different

- *What have I done and why did I do it?* – Guilt ALERT – you've tried many things before which led you down this path

- *I can't 'burp' properly what have I done?* – You have done nothing, your poor stomach now has a band wrapped around it. You'll get over it and learn how to 'burp'.

- *Why have I not been able to exercise the 'self-*

control' needed? – Poor me ALERT – accept it, move on

- *Why me, why did I need to have surgery?* – Poor me ALERT – why not you? There are, let's face it, other people in different boats with different diseases who may also be asking 'why me'.

This is your disease, now move forward looking ahead and not behind.

Enjoy today and each day for what it gives you ☺

I read a wonderful reflection and series of questions that I saved for myself to read on some of 'those days' when I doubted what I had done. Forgive me but I don't now know the author as I think it is anon. If I knew I would credit them.

'If'

If exercise alone worked then surely everyone would do this and never need to diet?

If diets alone worked surely everyone would be slim?

If psychology alone worked then surely everyone would have therapy and be slim?

If surgery alone worked then surely everyone would have surgery and be slim ?

So, at the end of the day there would only be exercise and none of the rest would be needed.

Tips on what to eat and drink post op

I guess you will expect a list of suggested foods here. Even a menu section. Sorry to disappoint you.

Your specialist team will give you a clear plan for the first few weeks. After that, it is a matter of trial, error and common sense.

You wouldn't try to get a king sized bed through small door without dismantling it so why try to push food or fluid through your band?

Common initial issues

- Not chewing = pain and possible blockage
- Eating too quickly = 'posseting'
- Eating too big a mouthful = possible pain and 'possetting'.

YOU are an expert on food.

Whatever you eat if you eat too much it is doubtful you will shrink as you desire.

Try to stick to calorie free fluids: water, tea and coffee made with skimmed milk. If you chose to drink juice, smoothies, shakes then it is unlikely that, in time you will shrink as you desire. If you eat junk food with no nutrients, or live on mashed potato (because it goes down) then you are likely to become poorly nourished, feel tired become constipated and possibly your skin will have a 'break out'.

Yes, of course, you could drink your meals and stick to soup or smoothies. Best way to get down more calories that are often high fat and carbohydrate.

Oddly, we were made with teeth. Soft sloppy or slidey foods are not what we were truly designed to survive on. I guess we would remain on mother's milk intake if this were the case! Anyway, this sort of food will 'whoosh' down, speed will mean that you are less likely to feel the volume effect of what you have had.

Work for your food like the hunter gatherers that we are. We may no longer have to 'hunt' for our food apart from shopping to buy it yet we must chew our food as did our ancestors. Remember the teeth of the 'Tolland Man?' and other similar. Teeth that were worn, 'fit for the purpose' for which they had been designed. Are your teeth used?

Yes you will take longer, as previously discussed. I want to hammer it home though, just in case you flicked over this bit before!

- When the meal takes longer, the hormones released that say 'stop you have had sufficient' are far more likely to have kicked in.

- After 20minutes ask yourself, 'do I really feel that I need to finish this?'.

- Am I eating this now because I like the **taste** and **want** to eat it all!

- Try to tune into your body, what is it trying to say to you.

- Pause or stop eating or drinking.

Like many others, I want to eat exactly what I want to eat and lose weight.

Along comes the personally loathed energy equation! I haven't got a unique or rare endocrine or genetic condition.

So, the bottom line remains the same. Even after surgery I won't lose weight if I put too many calories in! Our size and shape is directly related to how much we eat.

That familiar saying

~ Calories in have to equal calories out ~ it is true.

I STILL try fight this and struggle with accepting it but logically realise it must be true.

I think that all of us will try many techniques to try to slip those loved, 'little bits' of food, between our teeth without our bodies noticing!

Sometimes I try to kid myself that a whole tub of sour cream and chive dip lasted more than one evening. Almost wishing a lapse of memory, so I can avoid accepting responsibility for my,' hand to dip -dip to mouth -mouth to swallow', actions.

I'm not alone in this denial but it is a denial that can stop our weight loss post op at any stage.

See this email below:

> *Dear Sharon,*
>
> *I am hardly eating anything but am not losing weight. Is something wrong?*
>
>> *Sharon – can you write down what you have eaten today and let me have a 'squiz', may be something will become clearer*
>>
>> *Reply - coffee (latte 3), maltesers, quavers, bar of chocolate, home made gravy in a bowel with some potato, bowl of porridge, tea coffee and small fruit juice.*

Having sent this email back to me she realised what she was doing.

Growing up and accepting responsibility

We all have to 'own' what we eat. Sometimes, when we are eating to anaesthetise feelings or 'zone out' from the hard day at work we can literally forget what goes in. Log, learn and change your behaviours accordingly.

We don't have the Turks on our heels.

Typically, the Italians have such a wonderful turn of words when related to time.

The phrase above, of course means; 'We are in no hurry. No one is chasing us'

It will take TIME to change. Comparison is, 'truly odious' yet, many of us can tend to hold ourselves up to 'Cindy' who has lost 40kgs in a year.

Guess what, after 5 years both you and Cindy will probably have lost a similar amount. Does it matter what speed you do this at and if you do it the 'same' as Cindy? You are unique and your journey will also be unique.

How long did it take you to get fat? - I bet you didn't go to bed a size 10 and wake a size 30. How long will it therefore take to reduce? It doesn't matter. If the, size trend is down - that's a victory.

So, *'Piano Piano'* - 'Slowly slowly'. The Turks are not on our heels

Am I really hungry?

If you comfort eat it is likely you do it as there is no comfort available for you from elsewhere. It's normal to eat for emotional reasons. However, not mindlessly, day in and day out. Also not in as vast quantities as some of us can manage.

Airline food is, to me pretty grim. Yet when the meals are heating and the smell drifts through the cabin I too want to peel the red foil back to reveal some 'impressively titled' meal. I'm not at all hungry yet I eye my neighbour's meal and wonder if he has more than I have in my little portion.

In reality I now rarely eat in a plane. I prefer to reserve my limited intake to better quality, small portions eaten with space and relaxation.

Pavlov's dogs started to salivate when a bell rang. We are such complex beings at a neuro-chemical level we can seek food because our emotional bell rings.

Even postoperatively we face situations that disturb our emotional equilibrium. Remember these emotional quakes may, or may not be, size and shape related :-

- An argument
- Wearing some tights that are too short all day trying to 'hitch' them up again!

- A tense difficult meeting with the 'least favourite' manager
- The book order not appearing in time
- A sobbing, hysterical child
- The dustbin bag splitting just as you lift it into the wheelie bin
- A shirt label rubbing your neck all day, shoes rubbing
- Having your handbag or wallet stolen
- Losing your car keys
- Running late for an important meeting
- A death

Some of us have poor strategies to deal with what, for some, are quite normal challenges. Intellect has no relevance to this, understanding does.

I know, for example, as a stressed, working young mother I thought I was more than capable of being 'mother earth'. Outwardly I did a good job of being in control. I did so by having no time to myself, continual exhaustion, resulting depression and a growing ability to continually eat. This continual eating ability was simply in order to remain calm and maintain a 'numbness', a degree of anaesthesia from what was going on around me. 'Fridge cruising' being far more comfortable, and effective, than feeling reality itself.

With the above in mind could you try to listen to your basic emotions and body sensations; rather than wanting the effect of the food chemicals you choose to ingest.

Am I 'not empty'?

Instead of asking, 'am I hungry' ask yourself if you feel, 'not hungry'!

If you feel 'not hungry' that probably means you do not need fuel, food, liquid.

- You may need a hug!
- You may need a sleep.
- You may need a walk
- You may simply need a 5 minute break or some quality time to yourself.

I have recently started to watch a USA TV programme called 'The Dog Whisperer'. I sit enthralled by this man who turns dogs and their owner's lives around.

If he only knew that his dog psychology and wise words so often apply to me!

'Dogs live in the moment' - How true is that for me to remember when I think about my food and eating related behaviours.

This is even more relevant when eating with a band in

place. Am I living in the moment of food desire, or is this my true 'fuelling time'?

You know already that it takes about a minute for one mouthful to be chewed, swallowed, pass to the top pouch and then through to the lower stomach. If you are not seeking this slowed passage but are seeking instant gratification then stop because you are likely to cause a blockage, possibly vomit unchewed food.

Occult eating

The definition of 'Occult' includes 'Hidden from view; concealed'. As a verb it means to conceal or cause to disappear from view.

Do you recognise it? Do you recognise the power that rushed hidden eating holds? Take control and remove the power of occult eating.

If you want 'instant emotional gratification', with food then recognise that for what it is. Name it, even talk to it if you want to!!

Chose when and then eat solid food, sitting down to do so and take your time. Try to do this is a designated eating place rather than in secret, sitting on the loo, in a wardrobe, in your car or in the garage.

One of our biggest associated issues is that seeking emotional gratification we pile in soft sloppy foods rapidly, and often away form a designated eating place and usually standing or in the dark. This can gratify us with familiar resulting food/chemical reaction.

Eating between meals

I feel quite strongly that if you feel you need to eat between meals following weight loss surgerys then do so. However, are you eating for fuel or pleasure and taste? How are you going to eat sitting down or hidden and secretively?

If it is needed for energy – as with my son in law – then go for it. All Bites Count whether taken standing up, sitting down or lying down (as the Greeks and Romans). Alcohol and other liquids are included in 'bites'.

Banded or not, we all have the 'eat for England' type day. It is, as previously discussed, normal to eat for comfort, or seek chocolate at certain times of the month.

If you do it then OK, you have done it…… and so what. Remember it may be helpful if you open the biscuits in front of someone. Eat with them so the occult power and secrecy is removed or lessened.

Enjoy it, move on to the next day without the need to repeat it. It really isn't something you need to self flagellate over. Plan your next few days and move on without bringing the foil wrapped guilt with you.

Remember the Dog Whisperer – dogs live in the moment

but, with help, you can train them not to repeat unwanted behaviours.

It's OK to feel hunger

My son in law gets SO moody when he needs food. He is very able now to say – I need something to eat at whatever time of day. He recognises the feelings of hunger and we recognise the early mood changes. He fuels his body and then continues listening during the day to his clues and cues. At any time of the day he may choose to have bacon and egg, cheese on toast or a plate of 'left-overs'. Of course, some would say that he eats irregularly and between meals but who laid the rules out for his body?!

He works by his rules, listens to his body and it works for him. He is likely to eat smaller meals, rarely has 'seconds' and very rarely has dessert when he sits with the family.

I have learnt a great deal by Barny's eating and food related behaviours and I have tried to imitate or echo some of his approach.

Sally, a good friend, is slim, athletic and plays sport regularly – she even enjoys it!

When I ask her about what hunger is to her she told me that she likes the feeling of hunger. It is something she can control and something that she can relieve when she chooses to, and does so in a measured way. Then, when she chooses, it can go away.

Her meals are sparse in the day, generally she tends to eat late in the evening and is unconsciously conscious of how much, how and what she eats.

Food is a pleasure and a fuel but something she is actively involved with. Of course she eats in a social setting and of course she eats 'crapola' but not often as an emotional support. She also selects wholesome foodstuffs and shops only on a daily basis for meals.

Sally is one of the few people who has 'spoken' to me about understanding and learning to feel the feeling of hunger but not to be fearful or panic stricken. To control and almost relish the control rather than panic and shove anything in that I can to rid myself of something I call hunger.

There is always the exception to a rule. We all know the 20year old who eats junk all day and is as skinny as a rake but generally those who have a healthy, well rounded relationship with food and eating tend to be selective in what they eat.

They aim for quality and try new foods. If they eat a chocolate bar in the day they factor it in to their intake for the day and eat it consciously, often slowly or in parts but usually enjoy it for what it is – a food.

As bandies we hopefully learn, slowly, these skills and techniques.

Sleep

I love sleep. My mother says I have always loved sleep. I sometimes simply want to hibernate in sleep!

What I didn't realise is that sleep is so important to us. We burn more calories sleeping than sitting still watching television. No one seems to say what too much sleep is but I do know how grouchy I am if I get too little.

As a bandee please try to get enough sleep. If you are tired you're likely to pick to feed the need to 'keep going' so what about taking some time for you and schedule in some early nights.

Zzzzzzzzzzzzzzzzzzzzzzzzzzzzzzzzzzzzzzzzzzzzzzzzzzzzzzz

Urine

Urine, a valuable commodity for the Greeks and Romans collected and sold as a preparation for dyeing textiles. Later in history the salts left, after filtering and drying in the sun resulted in saltpetre. The primary use for which was gunpowder!

Sadly today we seem a little coy about the subject of urine. So, to be blunt is your urine clear?

If it is you are likely to be drinking adequate fluid for you. If it's mellow yellow or darker than that then drink water. Did you realise our bodies are over 70% liquid and we need to keep topping our tanks up. With calorie free fluids – Adams Ale – water!

Bowels

If we are shy about urine then we are definitely not Romanesque with bowel habits or consistency. No public and communal lavatories in the 2000's!

I'll keep it brief.

Your bowel is about 9metres long and a lot goes on in there. A normal stool should look a little like a sausage perhaps with cracks on the surface or smooth and soft. It is expected that someone can go to the loo once a day between 1 and 3 days.

Pre op you may 'do a poo' each time you go to the loo. We eat more and often continually when fat so our bowels respond but increasing the exit rates.

When you have had a band it is likely that you will have your bowels open far less frequently. However 1-3 days is acceptable.

If you are having your bowels open less than 3 times a week, have pain or your stools are hard and dry it is likely that you are constipated. You may also have bad breath, bad taste in your mouth feel more tired and even feel less hungry.

There are many possible causes for constipation (e.g. drugs, alcohol, disease, and even pregnancy!) you must always seek medical advice if you have a change of bowel habits or if you are concerned.

For the purposes of this part of the book I will say concentrate on Food types , Fluids and Activity .

Aim to keep your pooh soft and sausage like and you do this by keeping well hydrated and choosing food with fibre and that is unprocessed where possible. Check out http:// www.nhs.uk/LiveWell/Goodfood/Pages/Goodfoodhome. aspx for ideas.

Relationships, Sex life and Sexuality

Relationships

Dixon and O'Brien – two medics from Australia, have worked in the weight loss surgery world for many years. They are renowned for the quality and volume of associated research linked to gastric band patients.

It has been recognised, by many and for many years that a change in shape and size frequently places pressure on established relationships and partnerships. It may be that your 'significant other', feels safe, or prefers you to remain the shape and size you are and this may well place pressure on floundering (or established) relationships. Be aware.

Sex life

As an ex-midwife this subject was not uncommon and frequently came up for discussion. Oddly enough the same happens in bariatrics.

If you have been balancing on pillows for some years, or not really been enjoying this side of your life you may be surprised that, as you change shape, your sexual appetite may return with vengeance. It is not unknown for those who have been trying to 'get pregnant' to 'become pregnant' unexpectedly within a short time after banding. If you are OK with the idea OK, but if not, remember you are increasingly likely to conceive as you shrink.

Unfortunately, some find that as their skin begins to be losen they find themselves unattractive and unable to participate in any intimate times with their partner.

It is worth discussing with your GP if this is the case. Sometimes there are simple ideas that may help.

Sexuality

I have had many patients who, during or following their weight loss recognise that they have been struggling with their sexuality for many years. I can, typing this, think of 4 people who have 'come out' following weight loss. Their weight loss journey has been one journey and now they embark on another.

If you feel you are unique in feeling this way it may be advisable to seek advice from relevant organisations in your area.

Activity from now on

Increase your activity when YOU are ready. I'm not going to sing the virtues of exercise here because I am not the person to do it.

I attempt to climb on and off my Wii but the days I haven't been on it are more than the days I have!

I do enjoy yoga but apart from that I bow to your superiority, and in some ways envy you if you enjoy any active sports or hobbies that you do or intend to do.

What I will say is that it is a personal timing thing. Do you feel better about donning your swimming costume now or when you change shape a bit? Lycra now or lycra later?

Whatever it is for you that has stopped you then listen to it because you may be able to address your fears and start regular activity.

At the very beginning I would suggest to walk a house and back, then walk two houses and back and from then plan how far to walk that you know you can return from. Following spinal surgery in my 20's I was the cocky young woman sitting on a wall having felt very proud that I have walked to the shops but not factored in that I would have to walk back!

Exercise, Activity or whatever you want to call it can be gradually introduced when you are ready. Don't be too hard on yourself do you really need to book a place on the London marathon for next Spring?

First months.

You have learnt that feeling of 'learning to burp' again. You have probably moved on to food that you enjoy but is leaning towards being 'safe'. In other words you know it 'goes through' however are your teeth challenged?

Time to move out of your comfort zone. Start to explore foods that are more challenging to eat. Try foods that take time and chewing and include solid fruits and vegetables as well as fish or some meats. Compare and contrast with others who have a band.

'Can you 'do' strawberries?' Can you 'do' Apple crumble or just stewed apple? Can you do curry?

Your body has been shouting at you for years to take care of yourself and slow your eating down, now's your chance to do it. You HAVE to eat slowly or you are likely to have discomfort or regurgitate. Now is the time to take your fingers out of your ears so that you can hear yourself and the signals that your body will give to you.

You may make mistakes as do we all and this is how we learn.

You will develop very subtle signs of having had enough. These are whispers to you that you have had enough. If you ignore these then it is likely your body will SHOUT at you to stop and the shouting may not be pleasant.

A whisper of fullness is a yawn, runny eyes or nose, hiccoughs, deep breaths, shuddering (like a seagull with a fish going down tail first). Take some time to recognise what your body is doing and trying to say to you.

If you have been distracted from what is on your plate you have probably have lost interest in eating and need to stop. Give yourself permission to leave food and not to clean your plate.

If you ignore these then you will be SHOUTED at. You will start producing more saliva than you thought physically possible. You will have pain from your chest up, a mixture of pain, froth and slime will be trying to escape and eventually an unchewed lump of something may be 'orally delivered' in slime.

If you stop at the whisper then you won't have to experience being shouted at but you need to learn to listen for the whisper well in advance to avoid the shouting.

Expectations

Immediately after surgery is now … for the rest of your life.

For so many of us we have spent years separate from our bodies. We put something in our mouths may or may not chew, then swallow. A moment on the lips, a life time on the hips.

Now think seriously about what happens to food once it leaves the back of your throat. Where does it go to, what does food feel like as it travels down our gullet (oesophagus) to our stomachs.

It is easy to focus on taste and we have for years wanted to refresh the nice taste by another mouthful as soon as food leaves our mouths and our taste buds no longer taste it.

With a band it is so important to enjoy your eating and the food you choose.

Learn to link your head, mouth taste buds, throat, gullet and stomach together. You will work far more efficiently when working in harmony and not separately.

Where are you?

Are you working in harmony with your body or are you still slightly separate and not totally aware of what happens once you have swallowed?

How often, for example, do you wear a scarf around your neck? It never ceases to amaze me how many people come to see me wearing clothes that almost delineate where their bodies start and end. In some ways almost saying .... this is the cut off point, look at my face, my nice hair or make up but not below.

My mind, my head and what is below doesn't really belong to me – it isn't actually part of who I am. I don't need to think about 'that' part because it has nothing to do with my food and eating related behaviours.

Of course that is a huge generalisation but for me it has become an interesting observation.

As you sit reading this try to check where your body is. Where are your feet resting, where are your thighs touching, your shoulders and arms. Are you aware of your whole physical body?

Often, as fat people we are far from aware of specifics and are more aware of our shape, or size, being able to squeeze between e.g. a space between two cars.

This journey will mean that in time you will become more aware where your arms are resting, where the soles of your feet are and what parts of your bottom are touching the chair and the sides of the chair.

Does it matter, what relevance does it hold when you are only 'coming for weight loss surgery'?

The relevance is that you change as a whole and you learn that you can go into 'ordinary shops' for clothes. That you can push your shopping trolley between two cars and still get through. That you can lie on a single bed to read a bed time story with your children without having one leg on the floor and your bottom exposed. You learn to feel where food is as it travels down your gullet to your stomach and beyond.

You are a unique being who is closely linked to your body, mind and spirit. Try to learn to fully function and not function from instant oral gratification.

When you eat with thought you learn to feel your food and fluid descend into your stomach and enjoy a longer process of eating. You stop a few mouthfuls before you experience the pain that shouts 'STOP eating'.

You will realise that you are more in tune with what is going on and that eating is more than a taste or emptying your mouth ready for more it continues for a longer period of time and slowly you experience a new fullness that is not being overfull.

Hopefully you will learn that good and bad are meaningless terms and you will move to I learnt x today and I am pleased. Tomorrow is a new day and I intend to listen again.

It isn't a walk in the park and it is a normal behaviour to turn to food for comfort at times. Ask your thinner friends if they eat when they need a hug or some peace and escape. The difference being that they don't do it regularly.

I have had a band since 2000. Two weeks ago I was so angry and upset about something I ran a sprint to the nearest food hit I could get. I ate a custard doughnut, I ate an apple doughnut and was still angry. I then ate a fresh cream huge chocolate éclair and its sister from the box. I was still angry, and, I think by this time I was even more angry that in spite of all my usual numbing/release strategies I was still angry. So remaining at high on the Richter eating scale I was on a roll. My attempts to calm continued through an asparagus, runner bean, peas, corned beef and mustard tsunami nothing was dulling my now 'full on eatingquake'. My pouch was hurting, my stomach was hurting, I was hurting as the anger had started to turn to hurt. I had some chocolate and a low calorie lolly and had to lie on the floor as the pain of overeating was 'ouch' and very risky.

After a few 'after eatingquake shocks' I was, I realised still angry. The storm subsided, the 'after shocks' spaced and I started to look at the fall out following one of the biggest eating quakes I had had for a long time.

Do I feel bad? Nope. I do feel a bit silly that part of me still went into auto pilot and turned on the 'emergency' food will soothe switch. I wasn't physically hungry so the solution wasn't and would never have been, or will be, food.

What have I learnt? That I am still learning and a work in progress. Thank goodness, it would be so boring to be perfect!

What is different between 2000 and now? I can tell you freely about what happened. I don't feel I need to hide in a corner, feel shame and eat to try to rub it all better. It is what it is, a learning experience.

As you listen to the cues and clues of when you reach the point of 'no hunger' you will lose weight. I guess, as most, you will push it, try to 'beat the band', or eat that mouthful in one. Eventually you are likely to get the message, 'stop messing about' and succumb to learning your new way of life.

As you change in shape and size so you will feel disbelief, numbness, enthused, invigorated and 'alive'. There is a world of things out there that you may have 'always wanted to' but 'not been able to' because you've been too fat. Swimming, cycling, fishing, 'Wii fit' ,walking even venture out to evening classes or further education. Try not to push the enthusiasm to the brink be wise in your choices. Aqua fit is one thing and swimming the channel is quite another, so start slowly and work up.

Your scales are not your friend – they are likely to give you additional stress so steer clear. Don't weigh regularly but measure yourself.

Some people like to have goals to aim for e.g. when I am a

size x I will buy a bike. Personally I am still too impulsive to cope with set goals.

For me goals take forever and I rarely seem to reach them so I change them or forget them. Only you know how you are with such tactics. Work with what you know works for you.

Emotional journey

Expectations My expectations tend to vary. I really want to succeed - that's why I made the decision to be banded - but realise that success depends on my mental attitude. Whether I like it or not, put simply, my mental attitude governs what I put in my mouth. I'm also worried about failure; perhaps because I see banding as a last resort and if I can't make it work, I feel there's no hope left. On the other hand, this fear of failure may spur me on to make more effort. I'm at the beginning of a new phase and expect rough times but hope I'll develop coping strategies, be inventive and experiment in order to succeed, without becoming obsessive (boring and time consuming).

It would be great (and oh so easy) to settle into a simple, steady rhythm and lose weight consistently but, realistically, based on my previous track record, I don't expect this to happen! On the internet, I've followed the stories of people who have been banded. One in particular was a weekly diary showing weight loss/gain and a comment on how things were going each week. Perhaps following this has been my most valuable experience because it showed, how for some people, what a struggle it can be. Even though I've heard it many times, it made me truly believe that 'banding is not a magic cure'. Or as my fellow hospital bandee sums it up, "It really is a head game, though, isn't it?!"

Other effects of weight loss.

I guess most of us will know the positive effects but what are the negative ones?

Here are a few familiar ones that pop up in clinic pretty regularly. I have also experienced many of these.

Grief

Sometimes I feel that I am mourning. The grief of loosing someone close to you or an adored pet is not mocked or laughed at. For many weight loss surgery people there is an overwhelming sense of loss. Loss of a close relationship with food and eating as they have always done. Something they have always been able to turn to in times of need. This separation has been actively chosen and for some it involves guilt or 'what if' I had not done this.

Grief and loss is normal in our lives. How we deal with it is personal and variable.

As you read what is the most precious thing that you have

with you at the moment? Is it the silver locket you mother gave you, your wedding ring, your purse and all your cards or your car keys?

Now imagine that whatever that item or possession is has gone, been stolen, lost, simply can't find it or even damaged beyond repair. How do you feel? How will you react? What or who will you turn to for help?

Reactions to loss or grief is a normal reaction. People experience such a feeling of loss following weight loss surgery and can equally have similar thoughts feelings and behaviours as would be expected had you lost something, or someone, very precious to you. After all, for many of us, we have indeed lost or had to change our relationship with what may be for us a very close friend, comforter and partner i.e. food and eating. We now can't, however, turn to food to soothe or comfort ourselves as that itself may form part of our loss.

The process of grief and weight loss surgery

Grieving is complex and exhausting. I think it was C S Lewis who said 'no one tells you how exhausting grief is'.

Following banding it is often the fighting with and trying to, 'keep things the same' that people struggle with for some time.

As I said previously, in my heart of hearts, I want to lose weight but I also want to eat what I want to. I am simply not being realistic in that desire and I have had to learn to grieve some food over the years.

1) DENIAL

Sometime following weight loss surgery we reach a stage that may be triggered by stress, boredom, loneliness or other emotional events. We can try to convince ourselves that nothing has happened. We feel little change, our bodies are the same as before and the band isn't working.

The initial healing period is over and pretty much two weeks following surgery eating is not that dissimilar to how it was before. We can even try to re-enact behaviours or 'rituals' that we used to do with our beloved food.

Picking the roast chicken skin as we carve a roast, pop a bit of pork crackling in as we stand in the kitchen, or munching on a hot buttered toast dripping with thick butter because we 'fancy it'.

We try and tell ourselves that nothing has changed and can 'push' food through albeit difficult at times but may well come unstuck with our efforts of mindless rapid eating.

We cannot deny what has happened when a bit of 'something' 'gets stuck'. We have pain, discomfort and even regurgitation that shouts out to us, 'THINGS HAVE CHANGED'. Yet may be ...maybe if I try to eat this ....

maybe it will go through because there really is not change.

Wake up and smell the coffee! You simply cannot deny that things have and are changing.

2) ANGER

I have, in the early days, been very angry when my family were eating something I made and I wanted to eat but it would not 'go through'.

The more angry I got the tighter my band seemed to get and the I was less able to retain anything. All this over something quite simple like wanting a chip! Only one but I wanted it and threw my toys out of my emotional pram when it wouldn't go through!

Anger can manifest itself in many ways and we can (and do) blame everyone and anyone.

Bottom line is we asked and sought for wls to help us address our probable distorted relationship with food and eating. We can blame other people, our mother, father, 'upbringing' for making us fat in the beginning and in the immediate , we can very easily blame our spouse, the arguing children or our partners for eating too quickly.

We can try and try to eat and tell the family not to throw our food away as we go to the loo for the third time following trying the one small piece of salmon we'd been looking forward to all day.

We can even be angry with ourselves for needing, having, choosing weight loss surgery!

You know what - it is sad, it hurts and it is difficult to be denied what has served us so well for so many years as a possible friend, confidant or love. It's healthy to be angry. For many of us we will have to grieve a very special friend and relationship linked to food and eating and we will battle it all the way because, on some levels, we do not want to lose it or allow it to be less important.

3) BARGAINING

Oh how many times have I tried to bargain with a small piece of silicone that has no brain is totally inanimate and is around my stomach!!

Why oh why can I have a series of identical meals and yet know that each day will be a different eating day. Sometimes we are able to eat everything and the very next day with the same food we can eat nothing. I don't know but it doesn't take the 'I want it' away.

We can even bargain with soft sloppy slidy foods to hope they will soothe us in times of stress. If only I could whisk up a butterscotch instant milk pudding mix and know I could eat the whole thing. Just to help me deal with the irritating email I just received!

For some people they try even to bargain with God! If You let me eat this I WILL promise that I will not xyz ....

It is a painful reality to know that we consented to something that has an impact on our lives on a daily basis.

I think we have all had brief moments of ' if only I wasn't restricted I could eat ..' and for some they will have a phase of 'what have I done', if only I could turn the clock back so I can eat this xxx.

Actually I know many non banded people who would love to eat whatever they want, whenever they want. They have to make choice between an extra portion and being able to fit into their clothes. I know no one who can eat whatever they want in whatever volume and not notice a weight gain.

Hey ho reality hits again. More in than we need will equal increased size.

4) DEPRESSION

Many who come to us for initial assessment have been diagnosed with clinical depression.

In a few cases they may hope this go once they lose weight and feel better physically. This is not always the case and for some it is a sad reality that even as a size 12, or 30 inch waist, the world is still a difficult and at times cruel place to live in.

Weight loss surgery does not and cannot cure all evils or hurts. The only thing that can change is us.

If you have had weight loss surgery or are seriously thinking about making change or having surgery you have, or are, making a huge step towards instigating a change for YOU so WELL DONE YOU!

5) ACCEPTANCE

The final stage of grief – hurrah! You learn to 'actualise or accept the loss'.

I still long for an ice cold lager on a hot summer day but it is far less frequent and far less intense. I am able to grasp new energy new hopes and new goals. Goodness it takes a while but you will get there.

As with the grieving process, following the loss of a loved one, acceptance takes varied amounts of time. I know people who take weeks, months or even years but many realise that the food and eating related memories they have are not primarily about the food and eating but the people, the event or the place that contributed to the wonderful memories and rarely to the food itself.

Look to what you were celebrating when you had that 'wonderful meal at x'. Who were you with? What made you laugh? What made you cry? What happened when you felt overwhelmed with a feeling of love and being loved? Was it truly the Eggs Benedict or was it the people and memories around you?

I do believe that many weight loss surgery patients carry deep sorry with them. Call it grief if you wish. Some sorrow can simply be from needing surgery to help us. Some can be for the lost years, the years of not being able to sit on a swing with our children or walk alongside our partners or the loss of being a young active person in the familiar peer group activities as many of us were isolated or self isolating. In some ways grief and grieving enables us to accept what we have lost in our lives and what we have lost in our relationship with food and eating. In some ways grief helps us to move on and enjoy the newness of what we achieve through our change in shape and size.

There has to be an end for a new beginning.

Chapter 10

MAINTAINING WEIGHT LOSS

I am still learning this one and I honestly feel it is the most difficult part of my journey.

I have read numerous self help books laying out supposed thoughts or feelings that I may have had about my shape and size. How did these make me feel when I read them? Well, usually pretty helpless, disempowered and overwhelmed by the enormity of what I felt the situation to be. I had tried and tried over and over again and my previous learning had always been resulting failure ☹.

Writers in such books would ask, what to many may seem to be reasonable questions. They would ask things that may have included issues that resulted in my panic and despondency, e.g. Am I worried about being overweight?

Am I worried about my health or longevity? Do you feel low in mood, or suffer from low self-esteem because of your weight?

Of course I had, what a ridiculous series of questions. I woke every day and I was the one living my fat body 24/7 and all the personal and physical issues associated with that.

My personal fat mountain was one that seemed far too far above sea level to conquer.

In 2009 Ranulph Fiennes, at his third attempt, made it to the top of Everest. He had tried twice before. Twice he had had to turn back. Once, having a heart attack and the second was suffering from exhaustion. Finally he made it to the top.

He had great support from his Sherpa who encouraged him to move on urging him to touch the rock to draw strength. Fiennes said a pre prepared mantra 'Plod for ever'.

The challenge of making it to the top of Mt Everest forced him to behave in a way that his wife said, 'does not come to him naturally'. He had to be slow, careful, acknowledge his body and have patience.

This amazing 65 year old man has a fear of heights and gets vertigo looking down but when he got to the top he looked and was amazed at what he saw. "It was just like Fairyland".

I ran through the known 'motivation angle' many times:

- What are my reasons for change?
- What obstacles might get in/ or are getting in my way?
- Am I kind to me?

I have 'checked my lifestyle' trying to record my intake, activity and even logged a food diary with colours and stickers. Times, days, triggers of overeating, mood at time of eating and mood after eating – yep I had looked at that too.

I knew the calories, sins, points and fat content of a lot of what I ate. In some ways I considered myself a food number guru.

What worked for me? Truthfully, most things worked for as long as I lived within the boundaries. Therefore why did I keep failing?

My personal climb to the top of my Mt Everest had been life-long. I had no personal mantra. I had no preparation and no equipment to survive in the thin air at the top of my mountain.

I had aimed to lose weight, indeed I could lose weight but

to sustain it and not regain was my personal mountain peak. I didn't have the training or the skilled Sherpa to encourage me to 'touch the rocks' once I had completed the training.

Doubtlessly you have read of people who had had a gastric band or a gastric band and have regained most, if not all, of their weight lost. My belief is that the training may never have been offered and if offered we can, so often think it isn't relevant to us. So many of us think we can do it without the equipment, the Sherpa or the training.

Following any weight loss surgery the training and support needs to be life-long if we hope to maintain our new found shape and size the best we can

Training and how to maintain.

For everyone, fat or thin, there are many reasons why we eat and only a few of these may be linked to hunger. Eating and food is not about 'good food' v 'bad food', restricting food or depriving yourself.

For me I now live in a 'trade off' situation more often than not. I 'fancy' a biscuit, I eat a biscuit, I trade it for a spoonful of peas with butter.

Plan

To eat in a healthy, or in an instinctive way, is about eating with thought. In the same way that we wouldn't go on a walk over Dartmoor in the winter with only 'flip flops' so too we are constantly reminded that we need to plan what we eat for where we are and where we expect to be. Those places are both physical and emotional.

So many times I 'giggled' when people said to me 'eat close to nature and eat what is in local season'. I have had to eat my attitude to that philosophy. The more I have seen people do this the more I have seen their maintenance. Old words can be heard to be very 'boring' but there are many truths in them.

For interest try logging what food and fluid you have for 3 days. There are many www sites now that have facilities to do just this. You will be amazed at how amnesic your eating and drinking can be.

The one that my husband used to 'bash on about' was to plan my shopping and go with a list.

Oh how tedious when you have to go week after week and be limited to the list. Of how annoying that I can't 'break free' from the familiar items in my basket if I shop on line. I wanted to be 'naughty', the rebellious child. To buy two cream éclairs and scoop the cream from both with my tongue before peeling back the chocolate covering and then throwing away the choux pastry case. I wanted to hide the evidence before getting home and hope that no cream stains were obvious on the front of my jumper. He was 'spoiling it', spoiling my fun by saying be grown up and plan – how dare anyone do that with me and my food.

What was going on though with 'me' and food in this scenario ..... well that is for another story.

Planning is key – a well known saying by anon

'Failing to plan is planning to fail'

I have to admit that as a woman I wasn't always right on this one.

Chose and understand.

Understand what food is, how it works, what it contains.

What on earth relevance will that make to my maintaining a shape and size? !

Increasingly there is research based information that foodstuffs affect and impact on our mood and eating habits. A few years ago there were a few seemingly kooky people who bashed on about this sort of thing. I would sit eating my whipped dessert rather poo-pooing the idea as a means of continuing to eat whatever looked good and contained numbers that I had no idea what they meant.

There were a few brave souls who talked about 'sugar sensitivity', children having breakfast because it improved their performance. The press released the information and many of us chose to forget the signposts offered and bit further into e.g. what looked like a chocolate bar but if you looked at the ingredients on the back the first 4 ingredients were sugar in one form or another. A true plethora of 'ose'. Almost at the end of the ingredient list .... chocolate.

While some may chose to live on a daily intake of lemon curd sandwiches and fish fingers (yes I have met that person!!) We truly need to realise that no one food provides us with every nutrient that we need.

Many nutritional therapists argue that our 'lack' of nutrients will lead to cravings and often site lack of Magnesium leading to a chocolate craving as an example.

We need to eat a colourful and harmonious intake to meet the demands of our bodies and, more importantly our brain, if we are to remain healthy.

Portions & fluids

Let's be totally logical about this portion size issue.

We eat too much volume = we grow in size. Simple as simple can be - for those who have no issues with size and shape.

What if you are a grazer? I could, if I wished, still graze my way through about 2 days food in a few hours. Portion size has no bearing on a grazer because little pick of cheese or a finger dipped into the peanut butter as you pass the fridge simple does not count as a portion.

If stressed and eating to soothe ourselves then again those mouthfuls are not a portion so really don't matter.

A portion is when we sit down to eat our meal. Look at everyone else's plate and realise that our's is well balanced and a perfect size i.e. smaller than theirs! Pat on the back well done Sharon you are doing so well. So why are you getting a bit bigger – you hardly eat anything.

Yep you know the answer and I have read Jessie Ahroni email this ABC – All Bites Count.

Bearing in mind that the average size of a non operated stomach is approximately the size of your hand it becomes a little more clear that we only need a palm sized portion.

We will ALWAYS be able to eat more by overriding signals and signs.

Bottom line is your bottom will increase in dimension if you have more fuel than you need. Your choice.

I could now go on about the importance of monitoring calorie free fluid intake, recording protein intake and choosing good quality foods. However, surely as a fat or ex fat person you are already an expert on all this stuff?!

Activity & sleep

I joined the gym. I knew I could. When I was fat I went so now I am smaller I definitely should.

I paid £200 for the honour and I went..... three times... when the weather was lovely in the Spring and I could sit outside reading and drinking a latte.

What no one could appreciate is that I really do not enjoy the gym. I don't like sweating because it has strong reminders of existing as a fat person. I loathe the sweaty equipment and quite honestly only enjoy the sauna or steam room.

Am I ashamed, no because I am being honest and true which is more than I could do with food and eating in the past.

Activity and exercise comes in ,any forms. It may be simply sweeping the kitchen floor and then washing it.

I have spent several weekends visiting the local tip with bagfuls of rubbish I had collected. That was excellent exercise. My daughter and son in law have recently bought a run down house that is, in its shell like state, creating huge amounts of exercise.

So as much as lycra is good for some I am not one of those and admit to the fact I'd rather be gardening.

If you would like me to write the mantra of activity I

can have a go but please do not believe it comes from my heart.

It is recommended that we have a period of 30 minutes of vigorous exercise a day. Statistically it is said that to keep an exercise log means greater motivation.

Support

Again – not really 'me' because I chat far too much and the www provides me with the outlet to do so. However, it is recognised that people who regularly have support statistically maintain their loss for more than 5 years.

I am guessing that this may include, family, a personal trainer, counsellor, peer support etc

My own Maintenance – oh it's a bit of a slalom ride at times. Training to maintain so that I can cope with the heights of my personal mountain continues to be my personal hurdle.

I am fortunate as I have people around me who will encourage me, as a Sherpa.

I too need to be urged on by touching some of the rocks in my life and I recognise that this is for life.

So, as much as I really do not want to do any of these things I have to admit they are useful in training to maintain.

Chapter 11

BAND ADJUSTMENTS - YOUR QUESTIONS ANSWERED

What are "inflations, adjustments or "fills"?

'Inflations', 'adjustments' and 'fills' are the terms bandees and professionals use to describe the procedure in which fluid is injected into the band.

This is through the port located near the surface of the skin.

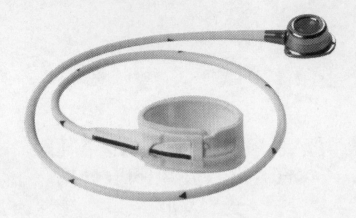

Gastric band (MIDband™) with inflation tube for fills and defills

What fluid is injected into the band?

Usually a sterile saline solution.

How much fluid is injected into the band at each inflation?

Adjustable gastric bands vary in total volume. This can vary from a total of 4mls to 14mls.

A tight band does not always mean good weight loss. Further inflations may be required over time and if you are receiving care. Privately then it is likely that you will be charged unless some are include as part of the initial package price.

Does it hurt?

Not usually. At most, patients report feeling a small pricking sensation similar to that experienced when giving blood.

If you have a needle phobia you can approach your GP and ask him to prescribe some anaesthetic cream. This is spread on the skin over your port area and covered with a clear adhesive film. Do this approximately an hour before your appointment.

What can I expect at a Consultation and adjustment appointment?

It is likely that you will 'bring' with you what you want to talk about. This should be an individual time to review the issues of celebration or concern.

If an adjustment is appropriate the practitioner can usually feel the port with the finger tips. Some may require an X-Ray.

A special needle is used to inject the appropriate amount of fluid via the port.

Once the band has been adjusted you may be asked to wait in the waiting room and have a drink.

This is to make sure that you are not going to have any significant problems liquid following your adjustment.

What can I expect after an inflation?

For a couple of days after the adjustment you may recognise and increased difficulty and the need to slow down your drinking and eating.

I advise fluids only for the rest of that day and the day after. The gradually introduce a normal well chewed food intake.

When will I have my first inflation?

Who knows ☺

Manufacturers guideline often advise no adjustment before 8 weeks post operatively. Others are less prescriptive.

Some people never need an adjustment to their band as they adjust other areas in their lives and do not rely on the band for their successes.

When will I have my subsequent inflation?

No one knows. This is very individual for each person.

Are you still losing weight? Have increased your activity? Have you reached a plateaux for three weeks or longer. Have you noted what you are eating and drinking for 3 days?

Then decide whether you need another adjustment and ask if you are unsure.

How do I know when I need another adjustment ?

It can be very difficult however, as mentioned above you may begin to think about it if you have stopped losing weight are starting to feel hungry are able to eat larger portions.

It seems to me, from experience, that the less you 'fiddle' with it the better the long term outcome.

A slower rate of band inflation seems to me to have better results for people. Rapid adjustments reaching a maximum inflation level quickly may lead to possible complications. There is a very fine line between being optimally inflated and over-filled.

If your band is overfilled/ too tight you risk adverse reactions and/or damaging the band.

How many adjustments will I need?

No one knows for definite. The volume, rate and total number of inflations vary considerably between individuals.

Is the band ever deflated?

It is fairly common for the band to be deflated.

Most commonly, the band is deflated when patients have been over-filled, prior to a general anaesthetic or long haul flight. Your band may also be deflated if you continue to lose weight after reaching a comfortable shape and size, during pregnancy or for certain medical treatments.

How do I know if my band is over-inflated?

If your band is 'too tight' you may not be able to keep food and liquids down, you may wake at night coughing or feeling you are drowning and you may get some acid in your throat. Having an overly tight band not only means that you are more likely to eat junk or soft sloppy foods that are high calorie.

Long term an over tight band may result in significant problems such as oesophageal dilation, pouch dilation or band slippage.

If you experience excessive vomiting or reflux please seek medical advice. It may be recommended that you have a small deflation to alleviate the symptoms.

Your adjustment

Ideally it is best to have an empty stomach when you have a 'fill. So, try not to eat or drink for 4-6 hours before your appointment.

Following your adjustment we can be tempted to 'test the

band' to see if it is working. Beware, if you do this you may cause some swelling which can result in difficulty in swallowing liquid.

Take it easy – it is not a race.

This is a journey and will be individual to you. Please try not to compare where you are with where others are

Does my band need an adjustment ?

There are several types of adjustment before having your band adjusted.

1. Adjust your eating –

    a. Eat more protein

    b. Reduce the volume you eat

    c. Drink more water

    d. Try to eat challenging foods that need chewing

    e. Avoid excess bread, pasta and rice

2. Adjust your physical activity.

3. Could you adjust your thinking - about food, eating and weighing

4. Could you adjust your behaviour?

    a. Eat different foods, stop picking, sit down to meals, eat more slowly, chew more, remove those last few trigger foods from the house, don't buy junk food.

5.   Lastly, if you have adjusted everything else then you could get your band adjusted.

When you get close to the size you want to be it is really important that you go through the stages above in order. A band that is too tight does not equal weight loss.

CONCLUSION

So have I reached my Shangri-La?

I guess I have intermittently been there in my dreams. In some ways an 'Avatar' type experience, real or not real ? I see no harm in dreams and enjoying them. I feel more at peace. OK so I have a changed shape and size however, I am equally aware that my shadows of obesity are standing in the wings.

I hope I have learnt to sit back and relax a little more. I admit to having fleeting fear of regain feelings and I guess that keeps me aware.

I live with my obesity at size 12 as do many others. The shadows and memories I doubt, and in some ways hope, will never go away.

Meanwhile I can enjoy today for what it is and if life gives me lemons I now try to chose to make lemonade and not sit looking at the lemons .... well some of the time!

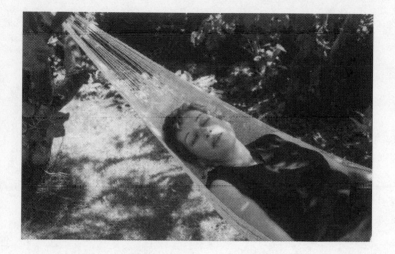

GLOSSARY

ABC

Alcohol

Alcohol has a high number of calories and also breaks down precious vitamins. It 'slips down a treat' and we don't feel 'full' with alcohol so it is something we can pretend is calorie free! A liquor on the lips can equally be a few inches on the hips – beware.

Addictive behaviour

There is an increasing belief that wls patients have an increased ability to 'swop' one 'addictive type behaviour' for another, shopping being one of these – so take care with your credit card !

Adjustment

Your band will have fluid added or removed throughout your banded journey. Sometimes the band may absorb fluid from the surrounding bodily fluid. This is not predictable and not frequent. However, if you feel a growing slow restriction of your band then contact you health practitioner.

Blockages

You will, at some stage get something 'stuck' or have a 'blockage'. We all do it and hopefully we learn by experience of pain and discomfort. It is not something to aim for so CHEW your food, and slow down.

Try not to panic. If something has 'got stuck' you will produce copious amounts of saliva and are likely to have considerable discomfort. Take some deep breaths and try to stay calm. If you get uptight it will make it feel worse.

Head slowly to the loo as what has gone down part way generally comes up or goes through but it may take a while for it to do so.

When something is stuck it may or may not be accompanied by pain or discomfort. If you some food and you always experience a block your body is telling you not to eat it again for a while. Don't write it off completely but try it in a different form e.g. chicken breast is often difficult for us but try different parts of a chicken such a thigh.

Annoyingly no matter how long you have a band or how experienced you may be it is highly likely that you will have something stuck from time to time. It usually happens when we are not concentrating, eating and talking, food cruising past 'pork cracking', a nibble of cake or 'only one peanut'. Simply put – don't eat on your feet and think when you eat.

Remember, what you can eat today, you may not necessarily be able to eat tomorrow, but you may be able to eat it the next day without problems. Presume nothing and take nothing for granted in this banded life.

If you can't drink any fluids it is essential that you seek advice. Do not let this continue for days. Dehydration is serious condition – avoid it.

Burping

Some people find that they need to 'learn how to burp again'. Once the band has been placed many people find that they cannot 'burp' in the same way as they used to and have to learn to do it in a new way.

Chewing

I cannot emphasise enough the need to chew your food until it is like baby food in consistency.

Constipation

You will hopefully reduce the volume of food you eat. It is therefore logical there will be less waste product to be evacuated.

If you have hard stools increase your calorie free fluid and fibre intake. If it persists then there are now several over the counter fibre supplements available that you may find helpful.

If difficulties do arise, discuss this with one of the team or your GP. A mild laxative may be suggested but do not use this as a first treatment of choice.

Cooking

Make use of thin gravies and reduced fat sauces with your meals. Miso soup or low calorie instant soup sachets made with ½ to ¾ the water amount specified make good sauces.

Some people find that vegetables need to be cooked a little more than usual and some vegetable are easier than others to 'get through'. Try steaming them just for a little bit longer. Equally meats that are dry or tough may be a challenge but a challenge is not a 'no' if you chew it really well

Chocolate

Chocolate rarely appears to 'get stuck', unless you eat too much too quickly and even then, somehow, it seems to have some arrangement going with the band so that it can slip past when and where others foods fear to tread!

If you really need it, eat it. You chose to have surgery, you may have paid a great deal of money to have an operation as a way to help you. No one is going to move in and hold your hand 24/7 or produce perfectly nutritionally balanced meals for you at every meal.

It is entirely your choice to eat what you so wish, when and how.

A 'flag up' though please don't expect your body to realise that you don't actually want to 'store' the chocolate as fat. Please don't expect a fat store amnesty – those calories are still going to be absorbed whether we like it or not. Your body cells haven't got the ability to sift or select which extra calories to absorb or not.

Denial

Are you honest with yourself? Do you know why you are fat? If you don't know why you are fat or if you believe you don't eat very much please seek some help in understanding. It is difficult to change if you don't understand what is contributing to sustaining the problem. Seek experienced help.

Do not eat quickly, if you find yourself doing this, put your knife, fork or spoon down and STOP EATING. Speedy swallowing and eating increases the chance of something getting 'stuck' – ouch!

Drink

Stick to calorie free liquids. A latte may be 175 or more calories two can be the same as a small meal but somehow we don't think of fluid as a meal – it can be!

Flaps

Flaps, Bingo wings, redundant skin, roman blind thighs, wobbly tummy – you may face the fact that when you reduce in size you may have to face 'empty', 'flappy' skin'. Loose skin versus rolls of fat …. hmmmm…… I know which I'd prefer. If you want to do something about it then seek some expert advice. If you have been an NHS patient the NHS may not be able to fund any reconstructive surgery. See plastic surgery.

Fills

Fills, inflations or adjustments this is when a special needle is passed through the skin into 'the port' that is placed just under the skin. Fluid is added or removed resulting in inflating/ tightening the band around the outside of the stomach. The process usually only takes a few minutes and uses no anaesthetic. Most people say it is virtually painless.

Rapid or over filling the band is theorised as a possible contributing factor to complications such as a 'slip' and / or damage to the band and/or stomach.

A 'fill' occasionally may result in problems. Immediately following a fill you may be able to easily drink fluids. However, that evening as you head towards bed you may find that you are less able to 'keep any fluid down' and are 'bringing back' white froth or are unable to keep your own saliva down. This can be a frightening experience. Some people experience this in their sleep, waking with a feeling similar to drowning as they are unable to retain any fluid and unable to relax into sleep without this happening again and again. You MUST contact your health practitioner for advice as soon as possible.

Before leaving clinic take time to sit and have a drink of water don't rush away following your appointment. If, after a few minutes on the road, you feel you want to be sick then go back to the clinic for advice, do not leave it.

After a fill we recommend that patients to have clear fluids for 24 hours and then fluids for the next 24 hours. This is to allow for any inflammation to dissipate.

General hints

A band seems "tighter" in the morning for many of us.

No one can fully explain this phenomenon and various explanations range from the usual release of stress hormone, lying down over night, change of water content in the body, tiredness etc etc. I am not aware of any substantive evidence in support of any such claims.

Some women have also noticed that the BAND feels tighter during menstruation. For most banded people excess stress or anxiety may also be a contributing factor.

Others report increased 'tightness' in: very hot weather, change of season, over tiredness, when taking some opiate based pain killers, flying long haul, smoking non tobacco substances.

These are very individual and some may experience no problems at all with these examples. You will find out what affects you.

Guilt

Why feel guilty if you've eaten something. Most people Slim people eat junk however they don't over eat on a daily basis and that's the difference.

Guilt, in the therapeutic world, is seen to be an emotion that is attachment to judgment. Who we place as our judge, or the one judging us, varies but may include ourselves, our partner, our parents, society, slim people, 'fit' people.

Are you measuring your worth or defining yourself by other

people's judgement, or your own judgement of you? Fat people are often significantly attached to 'being judged' or 'judgement' and as a result we use those judgements as an excuse or a way of distancing our personal accountability of inappropriate eating related behaviours, thoughts or feelings.

Lighten up on yourself you don't need to be so negative on yourself. See judgement.

Hiccoughs

These can be a sign that you have eaten enough – so stop eating or drinking!

Watering eyes, sniffing, yawning can all be gentle ways that your body is saying – I have had enough ~ I am full please stop! If you chose to continue you may well vomit as you will have over eaten. If this happens you're not listening to your body's signals. Try to practice this.

Inspiration

How long did it take you to get fat? No way did you go to bed thin and simply wake up fat! It took many years. It will also take time and effort to reduce in size – but you will if you work with your band not against it.

A band can be your best friend, but if you mistreat it can be your worst enemy. At the end of the day though, it is a small silicone belt that does very little but help us to stop and think. We have to do the stop, look and listen with our eating behaviours a band simply cannot do that.

Judgement

Fat people are very critical and judgmental of themselves. Lighten up! You are a baby in this journey and everything in life takes time to learn. Take time for yourself and start to realise that you are a nice person!

You don't have to be a 'certain' size and shape to be 'you' or to be a 'nice person'. See guilt.

Kick start

You may have lost weight on a pre op food intake plan. Don't panic if you don't lose more. This pre op weight loss was a kick start that resulted in the loss mainly of fluid and stored sugars and fats. If you stabilise you are now losing fat not stores. Well done!

Liquids

You should ALWAYS be able to drink and retain liquids.

If you can't then you need to seek medical advice.

Don't forget – no fizzy/carbonated drinks.

The majority of your fluid intake needs to be calorie free or virtually calorie free ~ tea, coffee, water. One milk shake can contain more calories then a meal but you can kid yourself it is calorie free because it is a liquid.

Alcoholic drinks and liquors e.g. creamy alcoholic drinks are also high in calories. Try to avoid high calorie dairy, or non-dairy smoothies. Also try to avoid drinks with artificial sweeteners or colourings in.

Just because it's a liquid doesn't mean you can forget that you have had it. Because you have a band doesn't mean you stop absorbing calories in liquid because they slip down easily and are swiftly forgotten.

Long haul flight

Many people find that flying long haul increases the 'tightness' that the band offers. This may be to the point of not being able to drink. Why not have a small 'defill' of your band for long haul flights so you are comfortable during the flight and when you arrive.

Medication

You should be able to continue to take prescribed medication. A pharmacist will be able to help you in knowing which drugs may or may not be taken in a crushed or liquid form.

If it is a drug that can be crushed then crush them between two teaspoons or in a pill crusher. You can then layer the crushed tablets on a teaspoon with e.g. jam, honey, yoghurt.

We advise patients to avoid taking aspirin (unless prescribed by a physician) and other non-steroidal anti-inflammatory pain killers. There is a chance that they may irritate the stomach and in some cases are thought to contribute to ulcers. Please discuss this with your GP

MRI

Many who have a band need to lose weight so that they can have other surgery e.g. hip or knee replacements.

MRI is a commonly used method to aid diagnosis and it is important that you find out if your port or banding system is safe in an MRI scanner. Most manufacturers have details available and you, or the radiologists are able to contact them to ask.

Nutrition

Fat people can be poorly nourished too! Get into the habit of taking a chewable multivitamin that your dietician recommends for you.

Eat a varied well balanced menu. PLAN in advance what, where and how you are going to eat your meal.

Enjoy each mouthful, chewing slowly and thoroughly until it is like a 'baby food' consistency.

Your dietician/nutritionist will be able to advise you but you will need to seek the advice. Gone are the days that these professionals will order you to 'do' a diet, not to 'xyz' or that you 'must' do something. The majority are highly skilled professionals and are able to help you on your behavioural change pathway.

Ongoing

Believe this journey is for life – a process.

Weight loss is not a destination it truly is a journey of self exploration and learning. It is most certainly not the quick fix option with a permanent outcome. It is challenging at all levels, scary at some, enlightening at others and has many facets of learning attached. If you don't work with it then you will be likely to have a very negative experience of it.

Pain

If you are experience unexpected pain and vomiting or, are unable to drink and fluids please seek experienced medical help.

Planning

"We don't have a plan, so nothing can go wrong." Spike Milligan.

We often start our banding journey with the simple goal of 'getting thin'

"Failing to plan is planning to fail." Alan Lakein.

There is growing evidence that planning all areas of personal life is a commonality among those who maintain body size and shape in the long term.

Plastic Surgery

It is not always the case that you will need, or want, to have reconstructive surgery (plastic surgery) following weight loss. If you do want to consider this try to wait for a while to maintain your loss and to reach a good place of nutrition. Give your skin and body time to recover from working so hard at loosing weight.

In the UK it is important to realise that Cosmetic Surgeons are not necessarily trained as plastic surgeons (reconstructive surgeons). Research web sites of professional bodies e.g. the BAPRAS http://www.bapras. org.uk/cms/Home/2/seo.htm

Port

The port is made of titanium or silicone and is placed just under the skin below the waist line.

Once the outside wound has healed (about 5 days after surgery) you may feel some tenderness but should not experience pain. If you feel pain make an appointment to see your practitioner.

Pregnancy

Your periods may become more regular when you lose weight and conception is more likely. Several of our patients have been taken by surprise by a positive pregnancy when they have previously been sub fertile.

During pregnancy the band can be loosened to ease discomfort as the baby grows. Once you have ceased breast feeding then the band may be made tighter again and your weight journey can be recommenced. Remember it is slower and harder to lose 2nd time around – so don't 'eat for two'

Questions

If you want to know the please ask – please don't presume any health practitioner is a mind reader. I would rather be asked than learn someone has been spending energy in anxiety.

Quality

You are worth good quality care and follow up.

Sadly as someone who was desperate to be smaller in size I would have done almost anything to achieve this. At the time I didn't realise what a potentially vulnerable target I was for services who simply seek to make a quick buck. Research carefully and don't rush in.

Recovery

Usually gastric bands are placed using 'key hole' surgery. This minimally invasive technique means that you will be home the same day or perhaps an overnight stay in hospital. Most patients decide to have about a week off work and are able to resume normal activities with ease.

Shoulder Tip Pain

Approximately 1:10 people experience 'Left hand shoulder tip pain' following such key hole procedures.

It is unusual if this pain has anything to do with your shoulder and is more likely to be due to irritation of the diaphragm caused by the carbon dioxide which is used to inflate the tummy for surgery. The body interprets this pain as coming from the shoulder tip. It generally settles after 24 - 72 hours. Some find that gentle exercise, a heat pad or simple pain killers, such as Paracetamol helps. Others find time alone is the healer.

Sleeping

Sleep heals and contributes to reduction in anxiety and stress levels. Recent studies seem to show that weight loss improves when a regular adequate sleep is achieved.

It may be worth thinking about how much sleep you get and how you may improve the quality of sleep that you get. As you lose weight your bed mattress may leave a 'dent of history' in it. Be mindful of the fact you may need a new mattress and in some cases new pillows.

Sleep Apnoea - Obstructive Sleep Apnoea [OSA]

The 'classic' patient with OSA is an overweight middle aged man. In reality this is not the case as it may affect all ages, weights and genders. Common symptoms are loud snoring and day time sleepiness. In some cases people will fall asleep during the day e.g. while in a conversation or other inappropriate times.

A specialist weight loss team will be familiar with OSA further and investigations will be arranged following initial assessment should it be suspected you have this condition.

In cases of OSA you must be aware that without treatment your driving license and insurance may be impacted. Research further e.g.

http://www.osaonline.com/
http://www.osaonline.com/questionnaire.asp

Socializing

As you change shape and size you may discover another world outside your own home e.g. Dancing, evening classes, book club, swimming and for some running

Stress

Stress, premenstrual tension, over tired, lack of time to yourself – all these 21Century things can, for some, lead to a feeling that the band is too tight. Try to 'chillax', hang lose and rest. May be your body is expressing something that you need to hear and do something about.

Support

I could not and cannot continue to walk my journey totally alone. You may be able to. I have been grateful for my counsellor, friends and family during my metamorphosis. You may not be the same ... you may be similar.

Targets (realistic)

"Piano,Piano" ~ slowly,slowly

Ten Rules

1. Are you eating only when you are in true need of fuel?

a. If you're not sure drink a large glass of water 250mls/ ½ pint) and wait.

2. Are you eating solid, not soft sloppy well chewed nutritious food?

3. Are you sitting down to eat?

4. Are you paying attention to your fuelling?

5. Are you paying attention to your food, and how you are eating and to those around you?

6. Are you eating s l o w l y ?

    a. Put your knife and fork down between mouthfuls and chew before you swallow.

    b. Take 20 to 30 minutes to finish a meal. Then stop. If you take longer you may be pushing food down with the weight of more food above. This can then mean food is squeezed through the pouch and you can eat more than you really need.

7. Are you taking small mouthfuls?

    a. You can check by using a tea spoon, chopsticks, cocktail fork or baby cutlery for one meal. You'll know then how 'big a bite' should be.

8. Are you chewing, chewing and chewing and ..chewing your food? Oh yes and chewing …...

9. Try to avoid fluid with food Drink ½ hr before and ½ hr after meals. If you have fluid and

food then you are able to wash more food through. More food equals less weight loss.

10. Are you stopping at the first whisper – a sniff, watering eyes, yawning = had enough Are you pushing volume of food until your body is shouting at you– pain, saliva etc. This is NOT the sensation you want. Avoid it.

11. Hungry = eat. Think you may be hungry = don't eat. Eating to stop getting hungry later = don't eat.

Too tight

Waking at night feeling as if you are 'drowning'? Unable to drink any fluid? Pain?

Seek medical attention/advice

Understand

Understand how the band works, where it is placed, what type of band you have, how much it 'holds' – become your 'personal professional'.

A band is designed to be a tool, a tool to soften or 'dim' your appetite. A tool that gives you help to control how, when and what you eat ~ you have to do the hard work and change your learnt behaviours.

Deemed as the 'thinking mans operation' in some

countries you have to 'think', plan and prepare with a band.

Vitamins and Supplements

We advise all our patients to take a multi vitamin each day. It is usual to get enough vitamins from a well balanced intake each day. Some teams will advise that you have blood tests each year to assess if you are getting enough vitamin B12, folic acid, and iron.

Vomiting

Excessive vomiting can lead to severe medical conditions. Seek advice.

There are many causes of nausea and vomiting. It may, or may not be associated with being banded. Vomiting when banded may contribute to inflammation, swelling and in some cases bleeding.

Please seek medical advice rather than leave it.

Weighing

PLEASE STOP weighing yourself so often ~ even get rid of the scales!

Weight loss surgery is not about weightloss! This is NOT

primarily a journey of weight loss by the scales of justice or injustice!

You've been there, got the tea shirt and the tape and proved that such boundaries and interpretation of success doesn't work.

What the scales say before and after going to the loo, leaning to the left or right, moving them from one end of the room to the other, on a half hourly, 8 hourly, daily or weekly basis is not relevant. Our bodies don't know we are looking for even numbers in a straight line going down in a pretty pattern.

Our bodies are too refined for such a crude measurement and weight is a crude method of measuring reduction of size and shape. Think 'general trend' not linear loss.

Write down all the reasons you thought you wanted to lose weight on a business sized flash card and keep it in your pocket. Every time you think of something new or experience something powerful you experience in your journey WRITE IT DOWN. If you are on the hunt for food comfort when you aren't physically hungry pull out the card and ask yourself some questions e.g.:

Which will give me the most pleasure or benefit me more in the long run? An ice-cream or being able to walk up the stairs?

X –ray

X-ray screening is sometimes used when adjusting a gastric band but not always.

If you present with symptoms that are not 'expected' then you may be advised to have an X-ray contrast swallow to assess the situation.

Yoghurt

Our team as that pre operatively you eat a yoghurt only diet for 7 – 10 days. This is to reduce the size of the liver so that the surgeons are able to access your stomach area more easily. Fat people tend to have fatter livers and this does not help surgery or the surgeons.

Eating a 'yoghurt only' diet will mean that the liver rapidly releases its stored sugars and the water that helps to store them. This aids surgery.

You may find that your team advise a different type of pre op intake but it is usually for the same intended outcome.

Zealous

Be enthusiastic, passionate, fervent and almost obsessive about the weight loss journey you have chosen. BUT try to have realistic expectations, be kind to yourself and don't look to weight loss alone as the final prize – it is PART of a more complex journey.

No one can do this but you and no piece of equipment can do it for you either. To win this race it takes commitment and hard work. You have to be enthusiastic and keep training.

It is for life so enjoy it!

THE END